"*Playing With Memory* is so much the surface, Linda Zimmer's book lays out valuable techniques for helping people suffering memory loss, so it is extremely useful for caregivers, professional or otherwise. Far more striking, however is the vividness of this particular woman, her failing mother, and the cast of characters peopling their world, including, especially, Toby, the apricot poodle therapy dog, not to mention the vibrant sense of West Virginia landscape and lore that suffuses these pages. Therapeutic theory and expertise are one thing, essential in themselves, but making the story come alive, that's a different gift, one that Zimmer has in spades. What a beautiful book, made to be cherished."

–LOUISE BERNIKOW
Author of *Bark If You Love Me*, and *Dreaming in Libro*

"Zimmer's captivating memoir is an artful and art-filled tapestry of what it takes to be a loving caregiver. In turns tender, funny, touching, and tough-as-nails, she marches us through the hallways of a modern-day nursing facility to meet its reluctant residents, including her rambunctious, rebellious mother, and then shows us what creative, artful play can do for the lonely heart."

–PAUL LALLY
Director/writer, *Mister Rogers' Neighborhood*

"*Playing with Memory* provides a glimpse at the real medicine needed for Alzheimer's Disease—immersion in the creative arts. When the past and future disappear, there is only the present moment, and that is best enjoyed through group connection and creative expression. Linda Zimmer talks the talk and walks the walk when it comes to engaging the residents of Elkins Rehabilitation & Care Center. She enters their reality and joins them in song, art, and humor, and appreciation for the unique human and inventive contributions of each."

−SALLY BAILEY, MFA, MSW, RDT, BCT
Professor, Kansas State University
Drama Therapy and Gerontology

"I enjoyed this book both personally and professionally. Personally, it is a heart-rending story. Professionally, it can be a valuable contribution to the discipline of medical narrative, which is used to teach medical students and other healthcare providers to understand disease states and unique treatment approaches."

−PHILLIP SCIBILIA, Ph.D.
Professor of Medical Humanities
Caspersen School of Graduate Studies, Drew University

"With wit, wisdom, and humor, Linda Zimmer has woven a memoir that is also a useful handbook for caregivers and families. Zimmer offers activities, songs, and solid research that anyone can use to help a loved one cope with memory loss and maintain emotional health."

−COLLEEN ANDERSON
Author of *Missing: Mrs. Cornblossom*
and *Bound Stone*

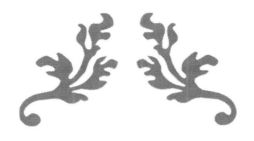

Playing

with

Memory

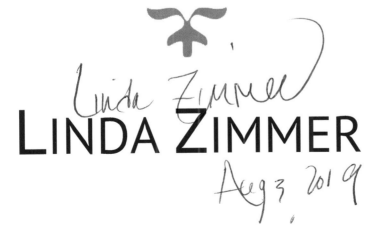

LINDA ZIMMER

Year of the Book
135 Glen Avenue
Glen Rock, PA 17327

I have tried to recreate events, locales, and conversations from my memories of them. In order to maintain anonymity in some instances I have changed the names of individuals and places, I may have changed identifying characteristics and details such as physical properties, occupations, and places of residence.

ISBN 13: 978-1-949150-19-3
ISBN 10: 1-949150-19-4

Library of Congress Control Number: 2018958234

Dedication

For my husband and my mother

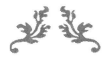

"If I had my life to live over again, I would have made a rule to read some poetry and listen to some music at least once every week, for perhaps the parts of my brain that are atrophied could have been kept active through use. The loss of these tastes is a loss of happiness and may possibly be injurious to the intellect and more probably to the moral character by enfeebling the emotional part of our nature."

—Charles Darwin, 1876

"Things change. If we can be happy with what we have now, we'll be alright, and I have the music!"

—Ellen Mc Cay Zimmer, 2009

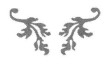

Introduction

Gentle Reader, this book reveals simple yet powerful tools and techniques designed to ease the pain and suffering of those with dementia and Alzheimer's disease, setting the stage for the players who depend on us as they maintain the ability to live productively and playfully in the moment.

Mise en Scène

(setting the stage)

Dramatis Personae (the Players)

At Blue Rock Farm:
>Linda
>Don
>Ellen

Dogs:
>Bootsie
>Tobermory (Toby)
>Django Reinhardt
>J. Jasper Jones

Cats:
>Peachy Wodehouse
>Jimmy (the big bopper)
>Lottie Lenya
>Ali Baba
>Louisa, Roly, and Poly – the Hemingway cats

Residents of the Elkins Rehabilitation & Care Center (in order of appearance):

Ruth	
Mr. Potter (aka Jimmy)	Nora
Ethel	Annie
Katie Mae	Georgia
Ruby	Paula
Sharon	Mr. Shannon (Sonny)
Estelle	Gladys

Chapter One

Somewhere Over the Rainbow / Stormy Weather

My heart is racing, open to the possibilities and promises of this sweet April morning. The path I'm on is more challenging than the circular high school track in Maryland where I used to run. The terrain here is hilly and unpredictable, forcing me to switch from my slow jog to a semi-brisk walk. But this is good; I have time to take in the view, which is vast now, as the trees are just beginning to reveal their buds and the tiniest shoots of pale chartreuse are emerging from the musky, mushroom-scented ground. Nature's first green is gold.

Because I'm alone on this narrow trail, I'm not concerned about impeding the progress of more athletic types. I'm ready to embrace peace and quiet. Peaceful maybe, but it's hardly silent here with the cacophony of early spring birds making their nesting and marital arrangements. But as my ears begin to separate the different calls and songs, I find it's not discordant. It's lovely. I move along, the morning symphony emboldening my pace and establishing a comfortable rhythm.

Wait... As I approach a bend in the trail, something crashes through the brush. I see a glimpse of white as a tall and powerful presence flashes past me; a runner appearing out of nowhere? I thought I was alone.

I laugh out loud as I remember where I am. I'm back home on our farm. It's my first full day here after joining my husband, who spent a frigid March in our tiny camper, unable to build the storage shed we needed for the building supplies we were hauling from Maryland.

We see what we expect to see. So, after five years in the Washington, D.C. suburbs exercising on a high school track, it's not surprising that seeing a powerful jogger in running shorts would seem more likely than encountering a white-tailed deer. The loud galumphing along the trail is in stark contrast to the graceful image presented in my imagination as deer ascend mountainsides or run through fields, apparently weightless. They are rather like the delicate ballerinas I've seen thundering onto the stage at Wolf Trap Center for Performing Arts, amazing me with the power of their delicate limbs.

This is my forever home, Blue Rock Farm, the constant love of my husband's life since 1974 when he first visited West Virginia and fell in love with the land on another April morning.

"West, by God" Virginia or "Almost Heaven" to geographically challenged John Denver. The Blue Ridge Mountains and Shenandoah River are not within our borders. Denver and the Washington, D.C.-based authors of the song must have been thinking about that other Virginia.

Perhaps influenced by the folksy charm of that very song and the availability of lots of cheap farmland, hippies flocked to the state in the mid-1970s and established several flourishing communes. After an initial wariness, these eager carpetbaggers and their new neighbors—the understandably suspicious descendants of the Scots Irish who settled this land— formed unlikely alliances that survive to this day. The communes are gone now, leaving many solid citizens in their wake, but although they may have lived the past fifty years of their lives here, raising families, serving on the school board, retiring now from legal, medical, business, or teaching careers, they remain outsiders. Just as my mother, Ellen—who moved to the mid-Ohio valley town of Parkersburg, West Virginia, with me and my father in the mid-1950s and spent the next thirty years as an elementary school teacher—remains a carpetbagger though her Scots Irish ancestry fits with the heritage of many in the state.

My husband Don's trajectory and my own are of course unique to us. For Don, the agrarian lifestyle was more than a political and philosophical choice. It's in his DNA. A Minnesota native, his parents were part of an earlier movement of back-to-the-landers after World War II, reading *Five Acres and Independence* and *The Have-More Plan*; the Olson Strawberry Nursery served as an inspiration for the Blue Rock Farm U-pick. While other homesteaders left their experiment with farming behind, Don's passion and respect for the land has only increased.

Like many restless West Virginians, I could not wait to "get the hell out of Dodge." After attending the state university, I moved to Pittsburgh as an actor/puppeteer and teaching artist. The siren call of West Virginia brought me back in the late '80s when I created a puppet therapy job at West Virginia

University and Don formalized his botanical expertise by completing a degree in landscape architecture. So, we found each other.

As our relationship deepened, Don explained that, despite a past marriage and other relationships, he was really "married to the farm." This line was a new one on me, teetering as I was on *forty is the new thirty* — the brink of middle age, with lots of dating experience in my portfolio. We'd go to the farm, about ninety miles from Morgantown, and I began falling in love too, with the man and the land. I harbored fond memories of time spent on my grandparent's farm in western Pennsylvania and because my theatrical training was always preparing me for a new wardrobe, I thought I'd look cute in wellies and bib overalls.

As a working puppeteer and a recently *educated* homesteader, we weren't exactly flush with the funds necessary to pay for improvements and support the dreams Don had for the farm. So, we headed for D.C., where Don worked as an increasingly in demand landscape designer. He noticed an ad in the *Washington Post* for a play therapist in a new children's hospital in Maryland and showed it to me.

"You can do that, can't you?" he asked.

"Sure!" I replied.

I had previously designed, built, and manipulated two dog mascot puppets: Sparkles, a friendly Pittsburgh-ese speaking golden retriever for Children's Hospital of Pittsburgh, and Jolly, a shaggy cheeseburger-eating crossbreed for West Virginia Universities Children's Hospital. Now Casey, a chocolate lab type critter with one white spot around his eye would become the centerpiece of the new pediatric play therapy program at Shady Grove Adventist Hospital.

Don and I both had rewarding work, but we were on a *five-year plan* to move back to our farm. Like the Hispanic workers on Don's landscape crews, we were hoarding our savings, living in a cramped townhouse and plotting our return to the *third-world state* of West Virginia, where outside interests had gone from strip mining to taking the tops off the mountains themselves.

The farm needed us to nurture her sugar maples, blueberries, and trout ponds.

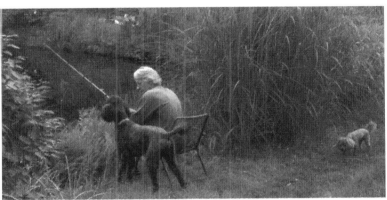

Figure 1: Don Olson fishing with poodles

We needed to build a proper house with studio space to pursue our varied artistic interests and provide a future home for my widowed mother, Ellen.

We began in the garden in April 1998. After all, we did have a roof over our heads, barely. The tiny mid-century modern, tagalong camper had received no glamping improvements while only costing the same as one month's rent in our Maryland townhouse. Although Don had lived in the decrepit structure that was the house on this hardscrabble farm, it was not

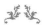

salvageable; we boldly bulldozed it and began rebuilding on the same site.

Amazing to me was that though temporarily abandoned, our farm offered us ramps (the native wild leek), rhubarb, and asparagus. The blueberry bushes had discarded their scarlet winter hue to reveal a soft pink budded promise of the brilliant, blue globes that would arrive promptly on the Fourth of July.

As a child, I loved the hymn "In the Garden." I didn't pick up on any religious significance. *"He walks with me and he talks with me"* was obviously written about me and my grandfather—him, the taciturn farmer, and me, the toddler who was doing all the talking.

So now, all these years later, I've got myself back to the garden, thrilled that we'll be able to grow at least some of our own food and open our blueberry bushes in a small U-pick operation. Did I mention I had no gardening skills? I like to admire, harvest, cook, and consume.

My mother, Ellen, was born on a small family farm in western Pennsylvania in April 1917, weighing in at three and one-half pounds on my grandmother's butter scale. Her twin brother was stillborn. She was then and always a survivor. A modern woman, she did not retain any of my grandmother's bread baking or chicken plucking skills; she moved on with the conveniences that were available to her. She is astonished to learn that I cook on a wood stove just like my grandmother. Frankly, so am I. My husband moved this charmer of a stove from his childhood home in Minnesota where his family occasionally used it for weekend breakfasts. The locals say that nothing tastes better than the food they remember cooked on one of these babies. Oh well, I augment it with a microwave and a toaster oven. The instant pot just being a twinkle in someone's eye.

By the end of the summer, our house is underway, the cats are settling in, I've found a job as a teaching artist in the county schools, and am utilizing the nearest library in the small village of Helvetia as my office. There is no internet access or cell phone service at Blue Rock Farm.

On my way home from my *office* one September afternoon, I'm startled to see a black standard poodle with a bad haircut leaping over the guardrail as I round one of the many hairpin turns. By the time I pull off the road, the dog is nowhere in sight. Babette, a black standard poodle, was my childhood companion. Wouldn't it be grand to have one again, a real dog, not a puppet dog? Bred as retrievers, there's nothing *froufrou* about poodles. They are ideal country dogs.

I jump out of the car as soon as I get home, hoping to have Don join me in tracking down the obviously lost, unkempt, black poodle.

He points out that I have probably just seen my first black bear.

I call my mother in Parkersburg to tell her the story, to laugh with her and to reminisce about Babette who died when I was in college. The Montgomery Ward's catalog was the only place we could find a standard poodle puppy in 1956 and she arrived at our train station in Parkersburg from Rhode Island on my tenth birthday, the passenger and freight railway systems being in place until the late 1960s. I call Mom frequently. She gives lip service to the idea of moving in with us and since we don't know exactly when our house will be finished, it's hard to make definite plans.

Lately there had been signs that her failings may be cognitive as well as physical.

"Where's Don this evening?" she asks.

"Mom, what do you mean?" I respond with some irritation. "Don't you remember he has that job as a night watchman at the coal plant, so he can spend days working on the house?"

"I'm sorry, honey, I forgot."

How could she forget? He's had the job for three months.

She calls three times in quick succession to ask me about a doctor's appointment that's been scheduled for weeks now.

Worried, I visit her. Her house is immaculate. She has a cleaning lady, a sparky woman in her seventies, who I think doesn't need the money, but has become devoted to helping Mom out. Mom spends a lot of time cleaning before Doris arrives and refuses to let her clean the bathroom. "No one should have to clean someone else's bathroom," she says. Mom always fixes a nice lunch and Doris provides the sweet tea. Still, it seems that *getting ready for Doris* is taking longer and longer.

I arrange for Meals on Wheels, which Mom shares with her dog, Bootsie. The mother I know would not have accepted food delivery any more than she would have had lunch at Bob Evans, "where only old people go." I'm grateful for her acceptance of this service because it provides another opportunity for someone to check in on her. The elderly delivery man always takes time to pet Bootsie and have a little chat.

Mom shows me a note in shaky handwriting, describing a special she watched on public television. It depicted an iconic episode when Fred and a young

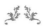

admirer in a wheelchair sing the song "It's You I Like" together (see Figure 1).

I had the honor and privilege of working with Fred Rogers on *Mister Rogers' Neighborhood*, where I created puppets and worked in the art department on set decoration and costume construction. Fred's playful and respectful approach to both children and adults, acknowledging the unique qualities of each individual, had a profound effect on me.

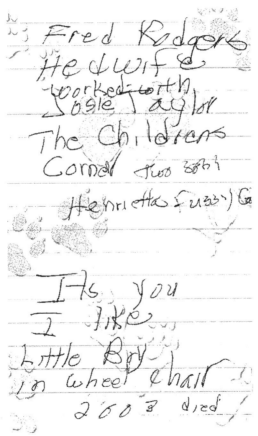

Figure 2: Ellen's handwritten note, 2005

13

Mom had always been proud of my work with Mr. Rogers and was able to be part of it. When I was working on the *Neighborhood* opera, "A Star for Kitty," Mom stenciled fabric for a bespoke cat bed—custom made—I was making for Betty, (Lady) Aberlin's cat character. Fabric shopping was even more fun when she helped me select dress material for puppet Betty Okanak Templeton and just the right faux leather for Old Goat in the production of "A Grandfather for Daniel" (Fred's puppet character: Daniel Striped Tiger).

I reflect further on Mom's handwriting. When had her perfect school-teacher calligraphy become so shaky? As we age, we lose some of our filters. This is sometimes seen as charming. "Old folks" can get away with saying the darnedest things. But Mom is being tactless and offending her few surviving friends with blunt comments and criticisms. "You really should tell Ed not to interrupt you when you're on the phone with me," she tells her friend Ruth. "Why is he always hovering around you, anyway? What do you mean, he won't drive you wherever you want to go? Ben [my father] was never like that."

When her minister asks how she's doing and whether there anything she needs, she responds with, "Well, all the lamps in my living room need rewiring." She's shocked when a bevy of church folk show up the next week to take on this and other household repairs.

"Linda, why are they doing this?" she asks.

"You said you needed help and they're helping," I reply, more than a little annoyed.

"I never said anything about needing help and I certainly don't need charity. Anyway, I have you to help me. You're my daughter."

"That's why we want you to move in with us," I interject for the umpteenth time.

"I will," she says. "But not now!"

I want my mother to be part of our lives and part of a carefully planned move, but inevitably, it's the phone call from her long-time neighbor—"Your mother has had a fall and is in the emergency room"—that sets our life on a new course. It will be weeks before she's able to make the move; hip replacement surgery is followed by physical therapy.

I spend time in my hometown alternating between packing up her house, my childhood home, for the move, and watching her struggle through the boot camp that is physical therapy. The hip fracture and surgery have left her vulnerable, confused, and in pain. She is not compliant with the physical therapist or the regimen of exercises that are designed to get her walking again. After the allotment of Medicare days is up, she will be released to the Elkins Rehabilitation & Care Center, thirty miles from our farm, for further therapy.

Don spends his time finishing the house and running Blue Rock Farm.

My contribution to my mother's care is limited; I'm the bearer of box after box of Crispy Crème donuts. They're not for Mom, who has no appetite, but for the nurses at the rehab center. I somehow think that this gesture might win her extra care and attention. It does.

I always carry a notebook, with contents I'm careful to obscure if any healthcare professional comes near, not because it's filled with insightful questions or observations. It holds sketches, lists, and an outline for a satirical puppet show with various costumed animals in a three-ring therapy room. I know that a family member with a notebook will also keep everyone on their toes.

In truth, I feel like I know nothing and I'm scared.

Having been a freckled free-range child of the '50s and a frenzied free-range woman for the next several decades, I've never been responsible for any living creatures except cats. I can see that Mom is going to need my protection and care. Without siblings or extended family, Blue Rock Farm will not be Walton's Mountain.

But somehow it works... for a while.

Don and I have planned for her to be part of our life. Without the resources of time or money to build a separate mother-in-law wing, Don has designed and built a beautiful home which, to my eyes, fits the site as perfectly as Frank Lloyd Wright's *Falling Water* fits its location in western Pennsylvania. Rebuilt on the site of the old house, it both hugs the ground and soars skyward, to provide studio space and a tiny bedroom for us, which Mom refers to as "the attic."

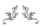

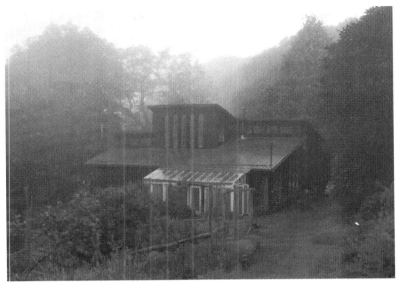

Figure 3: The house at Blue Rock Farm

The first-floor bedroom next to our common bathroom on the main floor is hers. No aesthetically unpleasing ramps or other devices designed to accommodate the elderly are in evidence. The solid cherry grab bars in the bathroom have been crafted from trees on our own land and look simply useful and pleasing. The front door is on the same level with the porch and driveway.

My mom and I have never been best friends. She's my mom. Although I was the long anticipated and cherished only child of my parents' marriage, I was never aware of being overprotected or spoiled. I have always been grateful for a childhood that provided me with the ability to entertain myself and perhaps internalize a *room of my own*. My parents seemed happy to let me be who I was and develop my life in my own way. They weren't happy that their young Republican turned into a Democrat when she hit college, but by then it was too late to establish parental control. Plus, they were busy with a new family member, my maternal grandmother.

So now I'm again in a family of three, juggling roles as wife, artist, and caregiver for my mother, who I will struggle to treat as the adult she is and not my child.

The age-related dementia that will become diagnosed as Alzheimer's, the most typical form of dementia, is limiting but not all bad. I will be spared political arguments between my husband and mother, now that Mom insists, "You can't really vote for any presidential candidate that you have not met personally." Does she believe that she had a personal connection with Ronald Reagan because she saw him in a motorcade creeping through downtown Parkersburg? Maybe she does, just as my grandmother believed she had a personal connection with Theodore Roosevelt who she saw on a visit he made to Uniontown, Pennsylvania; that other Roosevelt being, of course, beyond the pale.

Mom and I have mostly sidestepped politics and the great social issues of our day, to stay within the safe boundaries of the domestic arts, which for us includes music, fashion and decorating, pet care, and enjoying and preparing good food.

> *When all the world's a hopeless jumble*
> *and the raindrops tumble all around,*
> *heaven opens a magic lane,*
> *when all the clouds darken the highway,*
> *there's a rainbow highway*
> *leading from your window pane*
> *to a place behind the sun,*
> *just a step beyond the rain.*

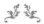

This seldom performed verse to "Somewhere Over the Rainbow" feels like an apt description of the terrain facing my mother as she moves to Blue Rock Farm and I struggle with new ways to open lines of communication. Abandoning reality, I attempt to enter her world, employing techniques of play and drama therapy. "Playing make-believe" is a rich memory from childhood and can be rediscovered to provide a safe environment to explore feelings and enjoy the moment. My years of experience as performer and creative arts specialist serve me well while I develop opportunities for us to be playful together: A Playful Protocol.

When involved in deep play, time stands still, and we are quintessentially alive and in the moment. Human beings, unlike most animals, never outgrow the ability to play. It is in fact a necessity if one is to maintain a sense of wonder and engagement in the world. I remembered Fred Rogers saying "the child is in me still, and sometimes not so still." The songs he wrote to help children cope with hopes, fears, and dreams took on new relevance as I strived for insights to help my mother and me find the joy and possibility of each new day. Even the titles of the songs provided understanding. I often found myself singing one of these as we went through our day:

"Many Ways To Say I Love You"
"What Do You Do With The Mad That You Feel?"
"Make Her Smile"
"It's You I Like"

As Mom's memories slip away I plan one last road trip to her childhood home in Pennsylvania. I want us to enjoy this time together, driving from Uniontown to Brownsville on the historic national road (Route 40) passing the Old Stone house built as an inn in 1817 and the place of my mother's birth in 1917, and spending the night at the Century Inn where both my grandmother and great grandmother had stayed.

Yet, I have concerns. Even the shortest trips to town for doctor's appointments or shopping leave me irritated by Mom's constant perusal of her image in the flip down mirror as she assesses and critiques her hair, makeup, and wrinkles. I don't look forward to a monologue on a four-hour drive. I prepare for the trip by obscuring the mirror with a picture of Sarah Jessica Parker, clipped from a magazine. I don't know what outcome I'm expecting. She will probably be annoyed or angry. Then I'll remove the picture. Surprisingly, she accepts the mirror's new occupant. Several times during our trip she checks the mirror, shrugs and proclaims, "She's still there."

She's still there... and so is my mother, Ellen McCay Zimmer. The problem is, I'm not sure which facets of her personality will emerge at any given moment. Who is she this time? The frightened former child? My devoted loving mother? My outrageously difficult and manipulative mother? The witty, creative second grade teacher? And of course, the many personas she's encompassed of which I knew nothing. I slowly learn it's better to be in the moment with her instead of trying to bring her back to reality. This is liberating for both of us.

Our best times together are when we're being playful, so we play. Playing with music, playing with art, playing with memory.

I find I'm not alarmed about having a second childhood. Not Shakespeare's *sans teeth, sans eyes, sans taste, sans everything*, but resuming the tumultuous journey of joy and discovery I remember from my own childhood, I welcome it. The truth is I've never given it up. Artists rarely do.

I'm just a kid again doing what I did again, singing a song. When the red red robin comes bob bob bobbin' along.

We play dress-up and shopping. I'm good at both. At first, we go to real stores, although shopping isn't as much fun as it used to be when I was a real little kid. Mom and I had always dressed up for downtown shopping which consisted mostly of window shopping, lay-away, and meeting my best friend Donna and her mother Fanny for lunch at the Wilmar Cafeteria or Stout's Drug Store with a real marble soda fountain à la Norman Rockwell.

On an afternoon outing six months later, Mom took off her blouse in the middle of the dress store in Elkins, instead of retreating to a fitting room, we opt for online shopping—which comes closer to my memories of downtown shopping anyway. We travel from website to website putting things in our shopping basket or adding them to our wish list. Real shopping had become exhausting. Online shopping is both relaxing and exhilarating. A worldwide market at our fingertips 24/7. Clothing, sofa slipcovers, pet toys, music, long lost items replaced on eBay.

I've always loved thrift store shopping. Before it became trendy, I had to disguise the provenance of any cool item I found for Mom there. Now when I bring something home and she asks where I bought it I can say, "A great new boutique... Goodwill!" If she wants to buy another or exchange for a different color or size, I say, "It's one of a kind, original, *couture*."

"And where did you get it?" she asks again.

"Do you know what a thrift store is, Mom?"

She would never have gone to one in the past.

"Oh yes, everyone goes there now," she says, displaying her new talent for responding to something she doesn't understand with a polite cliché.

We also enjoy dining out. One of our favorite destinations is Graceland.

Not *that* Graceland, but the former home of a United States Senator/timber baron who endowed a small private WV college at the turn of the last century. It's lovely for tea, dinner, or Sunday brunch. It looks like the elegant home of a wealthy family, which it was. I know the innkeeper and chef. They always tell Mom how nice she looks, how beautifully dressed. I'm so glad I scored the Valentino jacket at Goodwill. She's greeted warmly by everyone and if she decides to remove her dentures at the table? No worries. Wouldn't you look the other way if an elderly guest did something inappropriate at your own dinner table? Mom is surrounded by affection and warmth. She's happy.

We also go to *China*. While having dinner at one of the ubiquitous Chinese buffets in town, Mom asks "What's the name of this place?"

I vaguely remember glancing at the sign when we walked in. "Ah, China Maximus or Great Wall of China or…" My husband gives me the brevity-is-the-soul-of-wit look.

"China," I state boldly.

"Just China?" she asks

"That's right," I maintain.

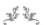

So now when we plan an evening out she often asks if we're going to China.

It's truly hard to beat the fresh produce, rainbow trout, and anti-oxidant rich blueberries on our own farm. But the occasional junk food outing can be good for the spirit. On a hot summer afternoon, we pass the Dairy Queen.

"How about a root beer float?" I ask. "You remember those." Mom smiles and nods. Does she remember? Oh, well. It's ice cream. What's not to like? We go through the drive-through. I order two root beer floats and a small ice cream for toy poodle Toby. Toby's order arrives first.

"He's getting ice cream," Mom shrieks.

"Don't worry," I reassure her. "Yours is coming. It has ice cream, too."

I may want to be a kid again, but am I prepared to be responsible for a toddler?

At home we can go to the theatre. I outfit a vintage suitcase with backdrops and find some old-fashioned paper dolls to serve as actors.

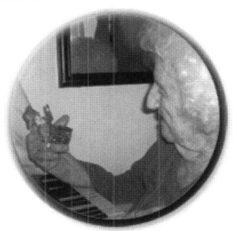

Figure 4: Ellen with finger puppet at the keyboard, 2006

We augment the cast with our own finger puppets. Thumbing through back issues of Vogue, we pick out the most elegant and outrageous creations for their costumes.

"Are you having fun?" Mom asks.

I am. This care giving, share giving is, well, kind of *like fun*.

"Like fun" is an expression Mom has always employed sarcastically.

"Take this pill. It will help with your arthritis pain," I say.

"Like fun," or "like fun it will!" she responds.

We are surrounded by fun loving critters. We play and cuddle with big poodle Django Reinhardt, toy poodle Tobermory, and all five cats. Mom brought her own cat Ali Baba and dog Bootsie into the mix and she's particularly fond of tomcat Jimmy, the big bopper. She says Jimmy is a cat you can really talk to.

We are inspired to write songs and poems about them, music being central to my Playful Protocol. It is the most consistent and successful communicator. Music encourages laughter, provides stimulation and relaxation. Morning hours are filled with satellite radio programming. Big Joe's Polka Hour and Mom's own piano playing are the fabric of afternoons. I play "John of Dreams" on the lap dulcimer in late day to help her face the dark side of being a child, the curtain closing on the day and sometimes ushering in nighttime terrors.

Mom has always made her own music and whether she's feeling elated, defeated, or simply lost and frustrated, she goes to the piano.

It can often provide the outlet communicated in Fred Rogers' song:

*What do you do with the mad that you feel
when you feel so mad you could fight?*

When annoyed with Don, me, or simply her new circumstances, she sits down at the piano. I'm so grateful that she can comfort herself through music. Her playing has been a part of my life for as long as I can remember. Because she can play by ear I was surprised to have her tell me about her years studying with her piano teacher. He encouraged her, when she was in her early twenties, to play in a local nightclub, but according to Mom my father persuaded her not to do it. "He was jealous of the piano teacher," she said. How fascinating. I didn't know any of this. Perhaps losing some of her filters is responsible for the sharing of stories once considered private.

I'm quite familiar with her repertoire, a mix of pop songs from the '40s and '50s, light classical, the odd Beatles' tune or a current country Top 40 number. The set rarely varies so I'm surprised to hear her playing something new one day, an unfamiliar melody with the refrain, *"After the rain the sun shines through. Bright sunny days for me and you."*

"What's that you're playing?" I shout down from my studio.

"Oh, just something I made up," she replies.

Two abilities remain with us for our entire lifespan. Even with a diagnosis of Alzheimer's, we retain access to our emotions and creativity.

Living in the country, for me, calls to mind this quote from Shakespeare's *As You Like It:*

And this our life, exempt from public haunt finds tongues in trees, books in the running brooks,

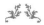

*sermons in stones, and good in everything. I
would not change it.*

Proximity to the natural world, organic food in
season or preserved from the summer garden,
loving family support, music, and pets. There are
days when I believe we are slowing the progression
of the Alzheimer's disease or at least making
accommodations.

Geographical isolation is not without its own
challenges, however. Weekly trips to town to buy
groceries and see friends have provided enough social
interaction for Don and me. Winters can be long but we
both have varied interests to stave off boredom. I build
marionettes and write puppet scripts. Don is
passionate about increasing his skills on guitar and
harmonica. We both enjoy reading and streaming
movies on Netflix.

But Mom requires more socialization. The rituals
of socializing remain and provide a sense of security as
other abilities decline and I wanted to honor and
support these. Her childhood memories were
grounded in community, not isolation. The McCay
family farm fronted on Route 40 in western
Pennsylvania. The historic road provided a regular
parade of automobiles in the '20s, '30s and '40s. Lee,
Noble, and McCay cousins filled the Old Stone house
with bustle and laughter during long summer visits.
Grandma McCay hosted quilting bees and a young
Ellen rode with her papa when he delivered eggs and
butter to the nearby coal camp of Brier Hill.

> "Mama, may I go with
> Papa to deliver the butter?
> As I anxiously awaited her
> answer, I could hear the
> spasmodic start and stop
> of the Model T. as Papa
> cranked and cranked the
> engine. From the accelerated
> sound I knew "Lizzie" had
> finally lurched forward,
> and was clattering to a
> stop by the side porch.
>   While Mama placed the
> freshly churned butter
> into "split" baskets. I happily
> anticipated the weekly trip
> to the mining town of
> Brier Hill, which was located
> in a valley, about a mile
> from our home in western
> Pennsylvania.
>   I was born in the old
> stone house which was built
> in 1817, and which had been

Figure 5: Ellen's handwriting from a school essay

I try to have people in for dinner a couple of times a month. In the summer, our blueberry customers provide a steady stream of visitors and Mom enjoys this. Winter, on the other hand, requires self-sufficiency and the ability to provide one's own entertainment.

More and more she refers to the farm as "Lonesome Valley." I point out we are in a hollow nestled in the mountains; elevation 3000 feet. "Alright, Lonesome Mountain, then," she says and heads to her room to watch *Big Joe's Polka Hour*. Thank God for Big Joe.

The sound of the walker comes on a Saturday night as Don and I are in the living room watching a movie. Mom plants the walker before us, blocking the TV screen.

"Don't you like good music?" she asks.

"Yes," we respond in unison. "That's why we're not watching Big Joe."

We all share a good laugh, which we need as tensions escalate.

Because she has no short-term memory, it's impossible to explain that I'm nearby, even if she can't see me. "Where are you going?" she demands to know. "I don't want to be left alone. If you leave, I'll get sick. I might even have a stroke and you won't care."

Two years pass quickly and slowly. I'm forced to admit that I can no longer provide a sanctuary for my mother. Her impairments, both physical and cognitive, have exceeded my ability to provide a safe environment. The closest skilled nursing facility (meaning one that accepts Medicare payments) is an hour from the farm. There, she would be safe from power outages and potential life-threatening conditions posed by winter storms. If a medical emergency would arise, she would only be five minutes from a hospital.

It's hard to know how I'll be able to infuse her life with the gifts of art and nature. These gifts have sustained her at Blue Rock Farm. I will seek out avenues to adapt The Playful Protocol to a new setting.

When I tell Mom, she needs the care available in a nursing home, she asks, "Why can't I stay with you?"

I respond by reminding her about her failing memory. I would have to be with her constantly to keep her safe. "You wouldn't want that."

"Oh yes, I would!" she responds.

A pause. We both break into laughter.

"Well, circumstances alter cases," she says philosophically.

Chapter Two

Someone to Watch Over Me

I s my mother's roommate alive or dead?

I see no movement from the bed by the window. An oxygen tank is visible and I'm aware of a hissing noise emanating from a specially ordered compression mattress. I move closer to the bed and peer over layers of beautifully embroidered linens which I recognize from my current obsession with *linen porn* catalogs as a probable 400-thread count. The sheets are embroidered with bluebirds and the monogrammed letter R (additional $6.00).

The bed's occupant is lying flat on her back, her unlined face capped with a freshly permed gray coif, carefully positioned on the contoured boudoir pillow. The mitted hand resting beside her clutches a soft cloth bearing the words "Sweet Thing." The hospital gown encasing the small form is not the regulation issue thin rag with small blue or gray print. No, it's obviously been made to order from soft cotton in a seasonal print.

As the first to arrive in this dorm-like room, she's scored the bed by the window which she will never be able to see. Her every need requires total assistance. There is a chair by the window for visitors. Tastefully framed hotel art adorns the walls and tightly arranged florist offerings sit soberly on the nightstand alongside hand sanitizers and boxes of latex gloves.

I lean in closer and her eyelids flutter open. She can hear. She cannot speak. Later, I learn she is responsive to music as I see her facial expressions change and soften as I sing and play the dulcimer.

"I see you've met mother." A friendly sounding, clear-toned greeting shoots over my shoulder.

I turn to see the daughter Lucy, a tanned, well-dressed woman in her early seventies, lots of diamonds, perfect French manicure, and expensive haircut.

"Mother and I are just country girls. We'll all get along great!" she says.

Is this the good match room assignment the social worker assured me she had arranged for us?

It's a disaster. Ruth's medical equipment takes up a considerable amount of the allotted space, leaving my mother in her newly acquired wheelchair, wedged in between the wall and the bed with just enough room for aids to bring in the odious lift that hoists her protesting body from the cramped chair to an awkward apparatus on wheels designed to make the trek to the bathroom and shower room.

It's a disaster.

Another woman enters the room, a large figure in lavender stretch pants carrying a package of chips and a 64-ounce container of Mountain Dew.

It's not a disaster.

This woman is a sitter, one of several salts of the earth, former nursing home workers employed by Lucy. They cover the day and evening shifts, feed Ruth the pureed version of nursing home cuisine, monitor her care, are on the lookout for slackers, and report back to their boss. They will also keep a concerned eye out for my mother.

Great! This eases my concern about Mom falling through the cracks and not being able to express her needs.

This is the same facility where Mom spent three weeks in physical therapy before moving to the farm. It seems to pass the tests I read about in books and online. While not fancy, it's homelike and this is key: it doesn't smell bad.

Do they have an adequate staff-to-patient ratio? Well... they have what the state requires.

The food will not be as healthy as what I could provide on the farm, but as an organic farmer and *locavore*, I realize my standards are unrealistic for an institution. When I request that whole wheat bread replace the ubiquitous slice of white bread (and yes, butter please, not margarine), I'm greeted by a blank stare from the dietician. She's not actually a dietician. As hospitality coordinator, she prepares monthly menus that are reviewed and approved by a dietician. She also orders the steady stream of sheet cakes that accompany every special event here in the nursing home.

The nursing home as we know it today came of age because of the New Deal legislation creating Social Security. Nursing home care could now be provided by the federal government. Previously many elderly people spent their golden years in county poor houses under shockingly bad conditions. While an obvious improvement, today's nursing homes have been described by some as the perfect marriage of hospital and poor house. Many, perhaps most of these facilities, do a good job of keeping people alive and safe, maintaining residents' weight, coordinating medications, and providing opportunities to promote mobility. But with the demographic of an ever older and sicker population, care falls short in the areas most critical to preserving quality of life—maintaining a sense of self and dignity as well as providing for opportunities to be creative members of society.

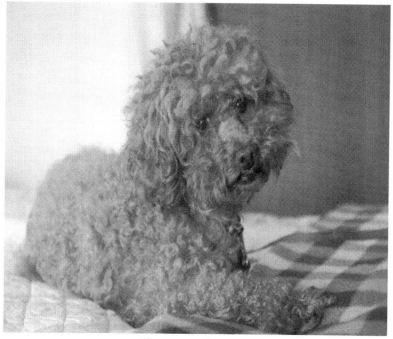

Figure 6: Toby, 2010

I plan to supplement the beading and bingo mentality in place here with steady infusions of The Playful Protocol: music, art, pets, humor, the modalities that have accompanied my mother on her good days and sustained her on her bad ones.

There is a piano available as well as a portable keyboard I buy to keep in Mom's room. We have art

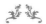

supplies. I'm close to a thrift store. Toby's visits are welcomed.

As a Creative Arts Specialist, I have the qualifications required to provide professional expressive arts services for the nursing home. This would be a new position in a facility which traditionally relied on an activity department to provide ancillary services. I present my case: The creative arts operate on a deeper level than arts and crafts, accessing problem-solving capabilities and providing profound satisfaction through a combination of physical, cognitive, and emotional skills.

In addition, I have one heck of a cute little dog.

I am hired as an Expressive Arts Therapist.

Chapter Three

How Much is that Doggie in the Window?

Everybody loves Toby. This toy poodle is ten pounds of sinewy body covered by springy apricot curls. Sometimes he offers a grin achieved by his one confirmation flaw: an underbite. Toby moved to our farm when his owner felt she was unable to give him enough time and attention. She knew we lived on a farm and were animal lovers. "What kind of dog is it?" I asked when she approached me.

"A toy poodle," she responded.

A toy poodle, a little dog. I've never had a little dog and think one wouldn't be right for country life. We already had a standard poodle, a big guy named Django Reinhardt, an elegant clown whom we adored. Standard poodles. They're the best!

Aren't they?

Maybe a poodle is a poodle. Mostly out of curiosity we agreed to meet him. He immediately filled a niche we didn't know existed, charming the cats and being welcomed by Django as the best possible tenth birthday present. At the local obedience school, the instructor suggests Toby possesses the temperament to be a good therapy dog. After passing the tests for certification, we began visiting a local assisted living facility. Now, he would partner with me at the nursing home, a full time working dog!

At the farm, Toby watches while I take one of his jackets or sweaters off a peg in the mudroom. He knows what this means. If I'm not quick enough, he will grab the garment in his mouth, shoot out the dog door, and wait for me by the Subaru Forester which I've dubbed the Tobster Roadster.

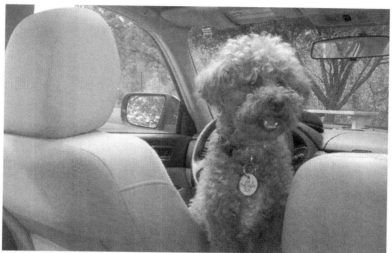

Figure 7: Toby heading for work in the Tobster Roadster, 2010

Once secured inside, he often naps during the forty-five minute to an hour drive (depending on coal truck and logging traffic). He's resting up for his job. Dogs need a job.

And work, he does!

His farm exuberance is curbed when he enters the doors of the nursing home, his bright yellow *I Am a Therapy Dog* credentials jingling against his collar and the Toby Zimmer-Olson name tag.

Traversing the length of the facility can take a while as we snake through yards of wheelchairs and walkers.

Outstretched hands wait to scratch behind his curly brown ears or lift him from the ground for a quick cuddle. One nattily dressed, dignified man seems particularly thrilled to see Toby. Seated each day at the entrance to the facility, he notes Toby's arrival and exclaims, "What a beautiful little dog! What's his name?"

I pause. "His name is Tobermory. We call him Toby."

"Toby? May I pet you, Toby?"

When we leave the building in a few minutes or hours later, it's a reprise: "What a beautiful dog. What's his name? May I pet him?"

Toby willingly, seemingly eagerly, has taken to sitting on residents' laps and nuzzling their faces. No matter how awkward the grip or unaccommodating the lap, he settles in as if there were no place in the world he would rather be. He does keep one eye open and an ear cocked in case there is a change in my itinerary.

Though trained, accredited, and well behaved, Toby is yet a visitor from the natural world—a world not much in evidence in the sterilized environment of the nursing home.

Theories abound promoting the benefits of being connected to nature. Hospital patients heal more quickly if their room has a view of the outdoors. Caring for plants and animals is also health promoting. To be able to touch, comfort, and, yes, love Toby, provides needed solace for those often bereft of friends and family. Rarely touched themselves or able to offer a caress to another, they eagerly accept this dog's love and trust. It is evident that Toby reminds many residents of their own loved and departed animal companions. I witness expressions of joy and sometimes a lingering sadness flickering across faces as they recall many beloved pets who have passed through their lives.

"He likes me. Toby really likes me," remarks a thrilled resident as Toby licks her hand, settling down on her lap.

One woman tells me the story of the family dinner table when her father would admonish them not to feed the pet collie scraps from the table. "Do you know what that dog did?" she asked with an unaccustomed twinkle in her eye. "He went around the table to my daddy's chair and sat there, quiet as a mouse."

"And did your father feed him from the table?" I asked.

"He sure did," she said laughing. "I'll never forget that."

Another woman talks about travels she and her husband took with their beloved beagle. When her husband died, she took Buddy to the funeral home to say goodbye.

But most of all, best of all, Toby brings them back to the present where they can live playfully in the moment. The past is forgotten, and the future can wait.

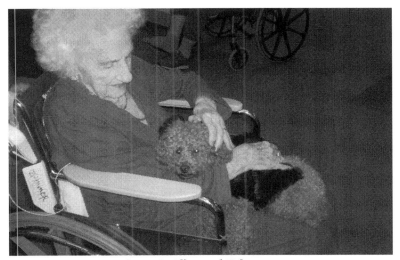

Figure 8: Ellen and Toby, 2013

I take out my mountain dulcimer and we sing familiar dog songs like "How Much is that Doggie in the Window" or "Where, Oh Where, Has My Little Dog Gone."

Then some new ones...

Toby's Song

(to the tune of "The Ballad of Davy Crockett")

Born on a mountain top in WV,
an apricot poodle, so very tiny.
He's had a great start now that he's four.
I really couldn't ask for anything more
Toby Tobermory, the one with the curly hair
Toby, Tobermory, he doesn't have a care.
Toby comes to visit, and you know the rest
You just say hello and he's sitting on your chest
He has a good heart, you know he's really smart
A visit from Toby will not be forgot

Toby the Snow Dog

(to the tune of "Stewball was a Racehorse")

O, Toby's a snow dog and I'm glad he is mine.
The wind's at his back. Snow's on his behind.
He dives into snow banks with the greatest of ease.
When it comes to his mission, he's aiming to please.
He has lots of friends here that he's eager to see.
It takes more than a snow storm to stop my Toby!

Just goes to show that a little doggerel verse can be grand!

Due to his own nature and careful training, Toby ignores the harsh sounds of buzzers and alarms while successfully dodging walkers and shuffling feet.

When his excellent nose detects the delectable aroma of food on a bedside table or perhaps something yummy dropped on the floor, the command: *"Leave it,"* puts him back on task. Although I can't allow the residents to feed Toby, I always let them know how much their visit has meant to him and leave them one of the Toby calling cards he carries in the pocket of his hoody.

Dogs love to work and Toby has found his calling. He also obviously wants to please and help me. When I hear the one loud insistent "WOOF" from Toby, I know that it's time to take a break or head back to the farm.

He's taking care of me. I am his human and his partner.

I visit with Toby in the communal areas, nurse's stations, sitting rooms, as well as individual rooms. When I take my dulcimer into the dining room, Toby holds court in the carpeted area outside the entrance, welcoming his friends as they come in for a meal.

One day, Toby and I are making rounds when we are cautioned by a nursing assistant not to go into Mr. Potter's room. "He's psychotic and verbally abusive. I wouldn't take Toby in there, Mr. Potter might hurt him."

We go in anyway. I begin by asking if I might play a song for him on my dulcimer. Perhaps caught off guard by this request, he agrees.

I begin playing and singing "Polly, Wolly Doodle." This tune seems familiar and now he notices Toby sitting patiently by my side. I suggest putting Toby on his lap while he listens to the music.

He accepts.

Carefully, I place Toby on the man's lap trying to keep his tail out of the Skoal spitting container attached to the wheelchair. As I launch into "I've Been Working on the Railroad," I notice Mr. Potter gently massaging Toby's curly body and humming along.

"You must have had dogs," I say. "You're so good with Toby."

"Yes, ma'am, hunting dogs."

"I bet they were your good buddies," I add.

"My favorite old dog, we used to lay down in the woods and take naps together."

After this initial visit I often leave Toby with Mr. Potter to dog-sit. I'm always nearby, but not in the room. If I stay, he tells me about the metal plate implanted in his head by aliens. He then instructs me to call the State Police or at the very least, bring him some "more chew." These requests are lost on Toby, so they simply snuggle while Mr. Potter hums softly in Toby's ear.

Once a month, the nursing home van takes a group of residents to the local art center for a noon-time concert. Toby is sometimes the bait to encourage a timid music lover to join the group. "I know it's something new and different," I say to Ethel, "but Toby will be there. You can hold him on your lap."

Ethel had a bad experience when attending a previous art center event featuring a mime—but hey, mimes can be scary. This incident forgotten, thanks to Toby, she climbs into the van with minimal assistance and enjoys a mime-free noon concert.

Toby provides a good focus for families when they visit their loved ones. It's sometimes difficult to find

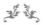

familiar conversational ground when residents are experiencing the fog of dementia and possibly forgetting familiar names, faces, and key elements of their personal histories.

I'd love to bring in one of our cats, but they are a conservative lot and don't want to leave the farm.

We have another standard poodle at Blue Rock Farm: J. Jasper Jones. Jasper is now the official dog in charge while Toby is at work. He watches us leave each morning and is waiting at the garden gate for our return.

The residents are interested in Toby's life and adventures at the farm. I tell them about the giant poodle Jasper, and even though he's not an official therapy dog, he makes the occasional visit. Far from being jealous, Toby relishes showing Jasper his other life. Jasper, another elegant clown, is greeted with delight by Toby's friends. His size allows him to walk up to a wheelchair and be petted. Like Toby, his town manners are on display as he keeps his loping and leaping behavior in check. I'm amazed at how he is remembered and inquired after even though his visits are infrequent. The residents quickly learn and enjoy singing "The Jasper Song" (to the tune of "Goodnight Irene"):

Jasper's a wonder dog
Jasper's a clown
You'll never have a dull moment,
when Jasper comes around.
Jasper lives in the country.
Sometimes he comes to town
(to get a haircut)
He's like a bull in a china shop,

until he settles down.
Jasper's best friend is Toby.
They're quite a sight to see.
Cause Toby can fit in your pocket
and Jasper's as big as a tree.

Toby figures prominently in art projects. By cutting dog pictures and phrases out of magazines, adding color with pastels, colored pencils, or acrylic paint, we make Toby collages. I make seasonal coloring pages of Toby as well.

I am astonished when people I don't know or perhaps don't remember meeting, stop me on the street or in a shop to inquire about Toby or pull up pictures on their phones of Toby and their loved ones. He has sat vigil with the dying and one floral tribute from a memorial service had Toby's picture attached to it.

Toby's a trouper, but I sense that he needs a space for respite and maybe I do, too. I have a lot of *baggage* in terms of materials I bring from my farm studio.

I decided to approach the administrator and ask for a space to store materials and provide a spot for my dog to take a breather.

"Well," she said sternly. "Space is at a premium. We have nothing."

No space. No money. No position for an arts therapist and yet, here I am.

I believe the administrator likes me—and more to the point, the positive responses my Playful Protocol has been eliciting from the residents.

She breaks the silence by asking, "What did you have in mind?"

"What about the closet in the activity room?" I ask.

"That's where we keep the folding chairs," she responds.

I try again. "What about the locked closet at the end of the classroom?"

"That's where we store the holiday decorations."

I recall one office I never see being used. "What about the big office by the gift shop?" I ask.

"Dr. Zirkle's office?" Dr. Zirkle is the little seen medical director of the facility.

"Yes."

I remember some hare-brained plan to keep kittens rescued by Dr. Zirkle's mother there. It didn't work out.

Toby's adorable upcycled suitcase bed would fit perfectly. "You see," I add, "Toby needs respite." Playing the Toby card is never a bad idea.

"Respite?" She looks confused and I'm beginning to be sorry I brought it up.

The administrator Denise is an intelligent, powerful, self-made woman. She started as a floor nurse in this very nursing home, put herself through graduate school and came back to run the place. An advocate for the elderly and children with autism, she is also a member of the state legislature. Her politics seem to be what I call a West Virginia Democrat (left-leaning Republican).

She's also, well, glamorous. She's created a mask-like persona that works for her: blonde hair, quite stylized, contrasts with lots of black clothing, expertly applied makeup, and a winning smile. This is a brand that serves her well as she poses for selfies with her constituents on Facebook. I believe I have seen behind the mask on occasion. Her face colors pink beneath the porcelain foundation when she speaks of subjects of deep personal concern. She even does wickedly funny impersonations in unguarded moments.

We have a few things in common. I do wickedly funny impersonations. I wear a lot of black and I have a standing appointment to have my hair foiled; and then there's Toby.

Denise loves Toby. She knows he provides as much therapy for the staff as he does for the residents. She has been known to bring Toby into her office and offer him a morsel of the state delicacy—pepperoni rolls—or a bite of her father's deer jerky. I may be a vegetarian, but my dog certainly isn't.

Although her door is always open, you must present your requests quickly before she's paged, takes a call, or loses interest in you and refocuses on her computer screen.

She's losing focus. She's taking a call from the governor. I pretend to be interested in something outside the window, avoiding eye contact and the signal to leave. I look up. She's back. I take a deep breath.

"About Toby," I continue as if she hadn't just been addressing important state business. I remind her that Toby clocks in more hours than the average therapy dog and needs to take a break during the day. This little guy has a sixty-minute commute and works twenty hours a week running his behind off as he tails me around the facility, never refusing to be jiggled, juggled, or jammed on a lap.

"Maybe you need a cabinet," she offers.

A cabinet? I think. A filing cabinet? Something to hold Toby?

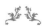

"And I want you to have something really nice," she says. "We'll order something. Thank you, darling." She dismisses me with the wave of a well-manicured hand.

A sleek black cabinet with shiny silver knobs arrives a few weeks later and is installed in the medical director's office.

As Denise says, "Doctor Zirkle is only here on Thursdays and he just wants to sit in my office and gossip anyway."

When a board member asks if she can use the office to store extra materials from the gift shop, Denise responds sharply, "No, that's Toby's office."

Chapter Four

Hey Good Lookin', What ya got cookin'?

As the morning sing-a-long runs down, clanging carts and swinging doors signal the arrival of the lunch trays. I change tempo and begin singing Hank William's "Hey Good Lookin'." I peruse today's menu for song cues.

"Mama's little baby loves shortnin', shortnin'. Mama's little baby loves shortnin' bread."

"Put on the skillet put on the lid."

"What do you suppose they put in the skillet today?" I ask. "Ramps, perhaps?"

"Ramps!" says Katie Mae. "Give me a mess of 'em. They're my spring tonic."

"Don't bring those smelly disgusting things anywhere near me," declares Ruby. "The teacher used to send a kid home if he'd been eating ramps," she continued.

I've learned the very mention of ramps—the native wild leeks—will energize and stir up passionate feelings about its consumption. Food is such a strong connector to our pasts and emotional memories. The ramp also signifies differences in socio-economic status. Country folks prized it as a spring tonic, but their citified counterparts objected to its strong and lingering aroma. Today it's celebrated in many local ramp festivals or "feeds" and given a place of honor on menus designed by hip young chefs.

Sharing memories of food, celebrating its place in our personal histories, is another way to bring the natural world into the nursing home.

I live on an organic farm, and sell maple syrup at the farmers market; I'm a foodie. I can't expect the food in the nursing home dining room to reflect my own taste and values. Still, I know that many of the residents grew their own food. I love to spark their memories and hear their stories.

"My grandma Lily made the best buttermilk," says Sharon, a resident, one day after listening to a story about churning butter.

"Grandma Lily?" another resident asked. "Wasn't her place over in Whitmer? I knew her. All us kids did. She always had something good for you to eat if you dropped by."

"Yes," says Sharon, "and that woman could make something out of nothing."

General laughter ensues at the acknowledgment of the resources of a farm woman. The nothing she had available was a well-stocked larder of preserved fruits and vegetables, a root cellar with potatoes and country hams, and a pantry with ingredients at the ready to whip up a batch of biscuits, cornbread, or cookies.

Oddly enough, because I cook on an antique, wood burning cook stove I can relate to stories about grandma Lily and her like. I have happy memories of my maternal grandmother baking sweet smelling homemade bread and cookies in her old-fashioned farm kitchen. For me it's a choice and I'm amused by the juxtaposition of the wood-fired cook stove and my computerized instant pot that awaits my command, providing a luxurious dinner in under twenty minutes. But I do love making maple scones and baking them in the wood cook stove. The results have garnered several blue ribbons at the Helvetia Community Fair.

Every so often we have apron days. I spread out my collection of vintage and antique aprons. Lacy Edwardian confections, sturdy calico and feed sack fabric aprons from the 1930s and '40s, novelty hostess aprons from the 1950s, and the chefs aprons I've crafted for myself to use in my own kitchen and on cooking days at the nursing home.

I bring in new yardage that I precut. The residents can hem this fabric and decorate with trims using fabric glue. It's not only women who respond to the aprons. Men remember their wives' and mothers' aprons. And what is a tool belt but another kind of shop apron?

Measuring, whisking, and pouring are all excellent means to keep small motor skills intact. Many of these moves are hardwired and come back to a resident who might initially say, "I can't do that." With a bowl and mixing spoon placed before them, kinesthetic memory kicks in. The hand remembers.

When we make maple syrup on the farm in early spring, I bring in some of the bounty to share with the residents and staff. While a pricey novelty to most folks these days, many of the residents remember making small quantities for family consumption. Labor intensive, then and now, it used to involve hanging buckets on trees and collecting sap on horseback to be cooked down in a wood-fired evaporator. It required about forty gallons of sap to produce a single gallon of syrup.

It still does, but on Blue Rock Farm the sap flows into the sugar house through plastic tubing aided by a vacuum pump and reverse osmosis machine. The sap is still boiled down over a large wood-fired, stainless steel evaporator. We may take advantage of modern technology, but the liquid gold provided by our sugar maples offers the same sweet flavor enjoyed since first discovered by native Americans.

One-hundred-year-old Marianne tasted our syrup and declared, "That's the way it's supposed to taste!"

By the spoonful or on homemade biscuits, everyone gets a sample.

Other favorites are corn bread, Irish soda bread, and pudding... we go for "instant" here—what one resident calls a "whip job." It can become the basis for a cream pie, fruit salad, and cookies.

After putting a recipe together and waiting for it to emerge from the oven, I read stories about food and family gatherings. I pass around the beautifully illustrated children's books of Cynthia Rylant and read excerpts from the Mitford novels of small town life by Jan Karon.

All five senses are engaged in these cooking activities and we have the tangible results of tasting and sharing the results of our efforts. Decorating hardboiled eggs, baking an Irish soda bread, pumpkin pie, or Christmas cookies are all good ways to connect to the change of seasons.

Although Toby is not allowed in the kitchen during the cooking sessions, everyone wants to include him in the fun. We sometimes plan a Toby tea party, make poodle-themed decorations, and invite him in for a morsel, and of course sing "The Toby Song." I bring a tea pot, tea cups, and seasonal flowers to put on the tables.

We celebrate birthdays by writing original birthday songs referencing the biography of the celebrant.

"Jenny, Jenny"
(to the tune of "Daisy, Daisy")

Jenny, Jenny, born in 1922.
When it comes to living,
she sure knows what to do!
Sewing, cooking and baking,
lots of yard work and raking.
Let's give a cheer.
We're glad you're here
We're wishing the best for you.

I was inspired to collaborate on these birthday songs by Mom who wrote this one for her next-door neighbor (see Figure 8 on following page).

Neighbors

For thirty some years
We've lived side by side
So there arent many secrets
We really can hide

We've both shared the loss
of someone we loved
But gone on with our lives
With some help from above

We've talked of our youth
of our lives on the farm
And are both thankful for
Parents who kept us from harm

Our teaching careers
We relive now and then
And are quick to agree
We'd do it again

There have been lonely days
And nights without end
But when the sun comes up
Were happy again

So today you are "ninety"
Please cherish the Day
With family and friends
Who have all come to say
"Happy Birthday"

Ellen

Figure 9: Ellen's handwritten poem to Evelyn, 2001

Chapter Five

I'm Your Puppet

Leaning in close to my Mom in her wheelchair, I can see that she's been feeding her stuffed cat some yogurt from this morning's breakfast tray. Kitty's well-worn, much loved face is stained a bright shade of fuchsia. Strawberry, maybe?

I take the hand puppet cat, Caroline and begin softly singing "Someone to Watch over Me" using Caroline's moveable mouth. Does Mom know this song? I can't remember her singing it or playing it on the piano.

Suddenly she sits up straight, makes eye contact with Caroline, winks, smiles, and joins in. Finishing on the beat, she gives Caroline a kiss on the nose and starts speaking in full sentences, which surprises me as she has been monosyllabic of late.

"You have two brown eyes, a pink nose and tongue and soft fur. I think you're a cat. How old are you? What do you like to eat? I'll get you something. You're going to have a nice life and learn how to do lots of things," she finishes.

This must be the way she encouraged the many young children who passed through her classroom over her thirty years as an elementary school teacher. And they were always "children" to my mother because "kids" are baby goats.

Although a puppeteer by profession, I initially hesitated to introduce puppets as part of my expressive arts programming in the nursing home. Perhaps because American culture unlike European and Asian cultures views puppetry as primarily entertainment for children, I did not want to appear patronizing or to seemingly treat the residents as though they were kids. There is a world of difference between *childlike* and *childish*.

I was already using music, writing, visual arts, and storytelling (all elements of puppetry) with my clients, so why not puppets? I was aware of the therapeutic power of puppetry for adults as well as children. Puppet shows are strongly visual, and emotion filled, making them natural communicators for people with dementia.

Puppetry is powerful theater and powerful therapy. I've watched as Russian puppet master Sergei Obratsov reduced an audience of adults to tears when he sang a lullaby to a simple hand puppet at the Kennedy Center. I've been on set at *Mister Rogers' Neighborhood* as actor Betty Aberlin had a quiet dignified scene with Daniel striped tiger—brought to life by Fred Rogers, accompanied by the melodic notes of Johnny Costa's jazz piano playing in the background. While a play therapist in children's hospitals, I created dog puppets who could serve as confidants for kids who needed to feel safe in expressing their concerns and fears.

A child's work is play. As it turns out adults, too, can use playful behavior to help understand and cope with new and troubling circumstances.

Before long, I brought on the puppets.

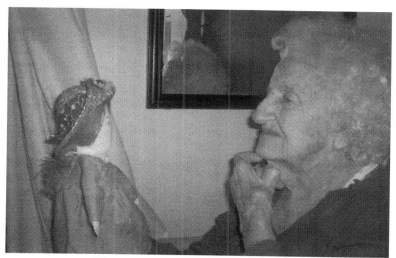

Figure 10: Ellen and puppet doll, 2010

The first thing I noticed is what's referred to in the theater as *the willing suspension of disbelief...* bringing in puppets without a stage, seemingly visible, yet invisible as residents interacted directly with the puppets. I introduced my own marionettes and hand puppets while acquiring a collection of Pelham marionettes on eBay and Etsy. These lightweight vintage figures were manufactured in England for children from the 1950s to the 1970s.

They are a perfect size to be operated by someone in a wheelchair and because they are string puppets, somewhat special and sophisticated. The distance from the strings to the puppets made for a magical transformation that captivated both the resident puppeteers and their nursing home audience. We made simple puppets, too. These stick, finger, and hand puppets could perform in the theater I fashioned from a vintage suitcase when Mom lived with us at the farm.

The puppets' very simplicity is what made them ideal communicators in the nursing home.

Residents are often approached by nursing assistants and visitors who speak rapidly and whose faces display a confusing array of emotions. The puppets freed the residents to explore a variety of emotions and story lines with shifts in time and place, transporting memories and imaginations to surprising landscapes filled with dramatic possibilities.

Sometimes I brought my own marionettes and puppets to perform for the residents. The Franklin and Eleanor Roosevelt marionettes were greeted with a delightful response from a woman who grew up in a new deal community in the 1930s.

"My brother danced with Eleanor Roosevelt when she came to dedicate Homestead School!" she exclaimed. "The Roosevelts did a lot for us here in West Virginia."

When Foxgloves were in bloom at the farm, I brought in an armful of blooms, dressing as Beatrix Potter and telling the story of Jemima Puddle duck, complete with fox and duck puppets (see Figure 10).

"Why, you're the woman whose stories I read to my children when they were young," said one enthusiastic audience member.

Because music and poetry are central to The Playful Protocol, it was a natural fit to create characters for "Daisy," "Take Me Out to the Ball Game," "Easter Parade," or "Stopping by the Woods on a Snowy Evening."

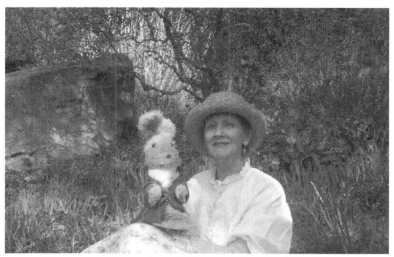

Figure 11: Linda as Beatrix Potter at Blue Rock Farm, 2017

The residents belonged to a generation where memorization of verse was part of the curriculum, and what's committed to memory at a young age is never forgotten. Poetry memorization was part of my education as well, so sharing my own favorites was pure joy.

I have a treasured memory of seeing two of my elder heroes who were not residents of the nursing home—Doris "Granny D" Haddock and Ken Hechler—reciting a poem together at an event in Morgantown, West Virginia, during the winter of 2000.

"Granny D" was a political activist from New Hampshire who decided to walk across the country when she was in her nineties to support campaign finance reform. Ken Hechler, a lifelong activist for the rights of coal miners, had been my congressman when I was a child. Haddock died at the age of 100 and Hechler at 103. They were kindred spirits who had obviously both memorized this poem celebrating the war heroes of World War I, as school children.

"In Flanders Field the poppies blow between the crosses row on row..."

How incredibly beautiful it was hearing them recite this emotionally powerful verse.

Inspired by that event, I decide to introduce poetry at the nursing home. My cat puppet Caroline becomes poetry Cat, puts on her poetry hat and we're off to the races. Her favorites are Edward Lear's "The Owl and the Pussycat" and William Butler Yeats' "The Cat and the Moon," both excellent choices for puppet shows.

Poets often celebrate nature. We revel in Robert Frost, Emily Dickinson, and William Wordsworth. Reading Wordsworth's poem about daffodils, *"I wandered lonely as a cloud that floats on high o'er vales and hills, when all at once I saw a crowd, a host of golden daffodils... and then my heart with pleasure fills, and dances with the daffodils,"* is a great way to let nature inspire us. We can go on to make flower puppets or become dancing daffodils ourselves with the addition of some shimmering yellow chiffon and spring-like music.

There's always room for a silly poem like "The Animal Fair:"

I went to the animal fair
the birds and the beasts were there.
The old baboon by the light of the moon
was combing his auburn hair.

I'm surprised when my mother recites a poem from memory called "I Like Beer." She doesn't, as far as I know. But what a delightful surprise to hear this.

Laughter is contagious and health promoting. It really can be the best medicine and something that is not lost with the onset of dementia. It lowers stress levels in the body by releasing endorphins creating natural pain relief. Laughter can make you more sociable in group settings.

As we work together making puppets, I listen to the residents' stories and learn about their lives. It doesn't matter if these puppet plays are completed. Sustaining an idea over time would be difficult for most residents. The pleasure comes instead from sharing our ideas and stories as we make the simple puppets. I often go home to my studio, work on story fragments, and reintroduce them the next day.

We all have stories to tell and it's important to listen as people give voice to the stories important to them.

Fred Rogers loved to say, "There is no one you couldn't love if you knew their story."

These are some of the residents' stories.

Estelle

Estelle Baroney is an enthusiastic participant in almost all the expressive arts programs I initiate. When I first met Estelle, the nursing home had not opened the memory care area. I sensed a newly displaced woman, elegant and terrified as if she had been catapulted from a safe, well-ordered life to an alien and confusing one. She drew me into her darkened room, perched on the edge of the bed and confided in me.

"I don't know why I'm here," she says in a whispery voice.

I reach for a folding chair propped by the dresser in her bleak, undecorated, private room, and then I sit down and wait for her to continue.

"I haven't been well, so maybe this is a hospital," she continues, slowly with precise diction and gentle dignity. "But now, today, I've been told Eddie, my husband—Mr. Baroney—is dead. It must be true, but I can scarcely believe it."

"I'm so sorry," I respond. She's clearly speaking her truth and whether he died last week as she seems to believe, or twenty years ago, doesn't matter. Her grief is fresh.

"Well, here I am, here I am. I must live here now. I guess that's that."

The next time I see her, a few weeks later, she's sitting contentedly in comfortable conversation with a gentleman, near the nurse's station. She's in control of her emotions now and shows a great deal of interest in the "pretty little dog" at my feet. I have my dulcimer with me and we sing: "She'll be Coming 'Round the Mountain" and "I've Been Working on the Railroad." Several residents join in the singing. Estelle seems to be forming a community.

When she moves to the memory care unit and we're making puppets together, she tells me more about Mr. Baroney, Eddie, the daring young man and his flying machine who stole her heart. Now I don't care what's real, I'm caught up in her story. She's a great storyteller, using wonderful voices to establish different characters—voices of her parents, Max and Goldie, and those of her siblings.

How old is Estelle? Sometimes she tells me she's seventy something. Other times she says, "Well, you know I'm in my nineties now." Always she tells me she's a leap-year baby. She is 93.

My own mother has always been fascinated by the exploits of Charles Lindbergh, the rock star aviator of her era. I think of this as Estelle tells stories about Eddie's adventures in early aviation. These stories which detail the different kinds of planes he flew, the places they lived together and their early days growing up in the mountains of West Virginia, maintain a certain consistency. One day Mr. Baroney said, *"Stella, let's go home, let's go back to West Virginia."* So they came home and after some brief period, Estelle got a phone call from a relative who delivered the message: "Eddie is dead." Estelle says he went out alone and must have had a heart attack, or she thinks he did. "Maybe," she opines, "he had a foreshadowing of his death," and wanted to get her back to West Virginia before he died. "Well, Mr. Baroney is gone. He's dancing with the angels," she laughs and adds, "...we think."

Estelle's personality and behavior does vary wildly depending on the time of day. Calm and pleasant early in the day while happily chatting with her gentleman friend or admiring Toby, she will storm the front desk by midafternoon demanding to know who's running the institution that she—Estelle Hall Baroney—owns and has generously donated to the community. She's most displeased with the management and she will either withdraw her funds or kill the administrator. Her usually clear, steel gray eyes are now rimmed red with anger.

Sun downing may be responsible for her agitation and outburst. This is the term coined to describe the disturbing behaviors that occur with dementia in late afternoon and into the night. The change of light, perhaps disrupting circadian rhythms, leads to heightened confusion, agitation, and aggression.

Because of the prevalence of this phenomena, I focus on quiet music and gentle storytelling in the afternoons. Rollicking sing-a-longs and puppet making are scheduled for earlier in the day.

Nora

Nora's vision is very poor. At one time an accomplished amateur painter she now becomes frustrated and angry with art projects. She is a lover of words, rhymes, and double entendre. She is also my mother's new roommate in the memory care unit. Although unable to see well enough to make or operate the puppets, she can give them voice through the many songs, poems, and silly voices she creates. I've become protective of Nora and enjoy having her sit near me in the puppet sessions.

While Fred Rogers kept inspirational quotes in his wallet, I keep slightly off-color limericks in mine. Writing my own private limericks about coworkers has provided me with satisfying short-term therapy. But in my wallet, I keep the classics:

> *On the chest of a barmaid at Yale*
> *was engraved the prices of ale*
> *and on her behind for the sake of the blind,*
> *was the same information in braille.*

After the activity aid delivers a stumbling monotone reading of some trite ditty in *Good Old Days* magazine, I enjoy taking out one of these politically incorrect treasures and sharing it with Nora.

Nora's daughter tells me she no longer shows any interest in making art. Although she did a delightful watercolor treatment of Toby when she was first in the nursing home, I realize that her diminishing abilities can now be a source of sadness, so I don't push her.

When Nora's daughter and niece visit, they are eager to show me pictures of Nora's paintings on their smartphones. "See what she used to be able to do!" they exclaim, as Nora sits silently nearby.

While I can empathize with their loss of the loved one they once knew, I try to get them to focus on her remaining abilities, to enjoy her quick wit and keen sense of humor. They are still living in the space where they quiz her and want her to remember facts that are lost to her.

"I'm going out to do some grocery shopping," her niece tells her one afternoon, "and I expect you to remember my name when I come back."

I attempt to redirect the conversation to include Nora, when they visit. "I bet you're familiar with Beatrix Potter and the wonderful watercolor illustrations she painted for her Peter Rabbit books and other stories," I say.

Nora nods and smiles.

"Well," I continue, "when I had the opportunity to see some of Potter's paintings at a Smithsonian exhibit a few years ago, I was amazed at how tiny they were. At one point she was no longer able to paint as she did as a young woman because of her diminished vision but she went on to become an avid gardener, creating amazing landscapes at Hilltop, her farm in England." I pause. "Do you like to garden, Nora?" I ask.

"Oh yes," replies Nora, with enthusiasm. "I love flowers!"

Lucky guess. When I can speak privately with her niece and daughter, I encourage them to focus on Nora's strengths and current interests, pointing out that we have a screened porch with gardening opportunities. Even with low vision, there are ways that Nora can participate.

"Oh yes, yes," they intone lifelessly, but their focus remains on Nora's inability to connect with them *in the old way*.

They leave, and Nora and I continue to find songs for the puppets as we work our way through *The Great American Songbook*.

Annie

Annie is a new resident who has not shown much interest in the various expressive arts programs. I hope to get her involved with puppet making or gardening because I've been told by her nieces that she was an avid seamstress and gardener. Because of her age and background, I ask if she planted a victory garden during World War II.

"I was in Baltimore during most of the war," she told me.

Amazingly, I learn that Annie, the youngest of five children, had never been off the family farm until responding to an advertisement in the local paper. She caught a ride into Elkins, West Virginia, and boarded a train to Washington, D.C., where she signed on with the Bendix Corporation to become a Rosie the Riveter, doing secret work developing radar systems used on military aircraft.

"They always checked our handbags when we went home at night," she said.

"Your work was top secret?" I ask.

"I was never able to talk about it," she said, and pantomimed pulling a zipper across her mouth. "Loose lips sink ships!"

"Now that would make quite a puppet show!" I say.

Annie loved being in the city, but as the youngest unmarried child in her family, she felt it was her duty to go back to West Virginia and take care of her parents. She later received a letter from the President thanking her for her important war work.

This fascinating information had not been mentioned by Annie's family, but they were happy to confirm its accuracy. I'm so grateful that she shared it. It was sometime later that I looked carefully at her last name and realized we shared a connection: When Annie and her widowed mother were too old to stay on the family farm, they sold it to a young man from Minnesota—my husband, Don Olson.

Georgia

When I meet Georgia, we comfortably fall into a discussion of our names and songs associated with them. Hers, of course, is "Georgia On My Mind." Mine is "A Linda Song." Georgia has no short-term memory, so although Toby and I see her several times a week, I am always meeting her for the first time.

We sing our name songs: *"When I go to sleep I never count sheep, I count all the charms about Linda,"* then, *"Just an old sweet song keeps Georgia on my mind."* She also learns "Toby's Song."

One morning I enter the communal area to find Georgia visibly distressed and agitated. She is usually content and philosophical about her lack of memory. But not today.

"I don't know who I am or why I'm here!" Her voice is laced with distress and desperation. "I've heard of amnesia. Do I have that?" she implores as I approach her.

"We've met," I say. "We know some of the same songs." I start singing "Toby's Song" and she joins me, word perfect. Next, we sing "Amazing Grace" then join hands and walk down the hall together. She's calm now as we enter her room.

"Oh, there's my bear and my pink tennis shoes. I'm home now."

Although she doesn't have visitors, I've learned that her family had a traveling band performing in local churches. I don't think she was in the band, as she has a hard time staying on key. But who cares? She sings now with abandon and always finds the words.

Chapter Six

In the Garden

"I come to the garden alone while the dew is still on the roses." I took these words from the old hymn literally when I was a child. What could be more wonderful than the garden where I walked and talked with my grandparents?

Connecting with the natural world is key to our health and wellbeing and being aware of the changing seasons is grounding. This can be challenging in an institutional setting. I bring flowers and blooming branches from the farm in spring and summer, autumn leaves in the fall, and pine cones in the winter. Touching and smelling these items trigger reminiscences.

The seed catalogues fill our mailbox at the farm beginning in early January. I bring them to the nursing home where we pour over them, picking out our favorites.

"One year, I went crazy and planted petunias everywhere," said Paula. "Even by the outhouse!"

I notice the phrase "I went crazy" used to describe what I would call the creative process. I like this. The second definition of *crazy* in Webster's Dictionary is: *"passionately enthusiastic."*

We begin to put together words and images reminding us of spring and summer. Using the seed catalogs as inspiration, we apply fabric paint and watercolors on muslin. I help them cut out the shapes and secure them with iron on fusible backing to create a fabric wall hanging.

Using the word images, I've collected. I compose this song:

Bloom and Sing

As I sit and wait for Spring
I think of things that bloom and sing
Wish for blossoms sweet and new.
Birds that chirp and peepers, too.
Roses blooming 'round my door.
Then I couldn't ask for more.
Here I sit among my friends,
singing songs of Winter's end.
As I sing, I know it's true,
Spring can live inside of you.

The song "Bloom and Sing" is added to the ERCC glee club repertoire.

It used to be thought that we were unable to learn new material after a certain age and that certainly we would not be able to grow new brain cells. Knowing this theory has been debunked, I'm not surprised when residents not only recall old familiar tunes but can learn new ones.

The nursing home grounds have curb appeal, with a landscaping company on retainer to provide seasonal plantings. Few residents can take advantage of these views. I was approached by an apologetic family member whose mother could not resist the urge to pick one of the pansies lining the entrance walkway.

Adorning our houses with flowers is something many people remember and enjoy so I plant an old-fashioned cutting garden, "Toby's Garden," and encourage residents to pick bouquets of annuals for their rooms.

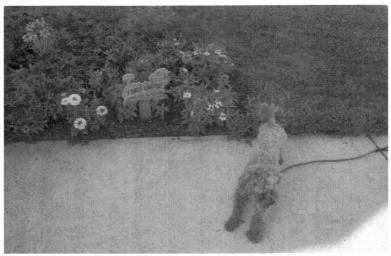

Figure 12: Toby in his garden, 2012

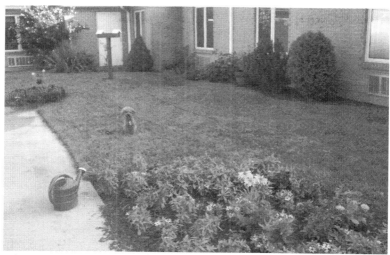

Figure 13: Toby's garden sits in view of some residents' windows, 2012

Chapter Seven

All God's Critters Got a Place in the Choir

As I describe the various creative arts modalities I'm struck by how music is part of all of them. Whether polishing off corn bread, playing with a poodle, puttering in the garden, performing with puppets or practicing poetry, music is always there. We are a musical species and music is a huge part of our emotional memory.

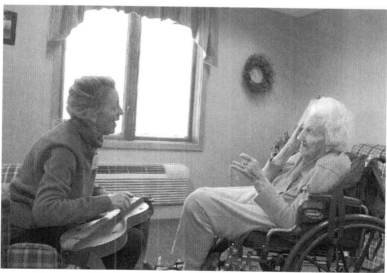

Figure 14: Playing the dulcimer and singing with Mom, 2014.
Photo by Jean Snedegar.

Scientists now point out that singing can boost your immune system by decreasing the levels of the stress hormone, cortisol, in the blood stream.

In Mom's early days in the nursing home, I bemoaned the fact that she could not always have access to her music. I would leave her with a portable CD player and headphones, knowing that the music would end before I got back to the farm with little assurance that a staff member would restart it for her.

One day while listening to NPR I heard an interview with Dan Cohen, the social worker who started the national Music & Memory program. Dan had great technical expertise as well as growing concerns about the isolation of his nursing home clients. He thought about how he would feel living in an institution being separated from his own music.

The design of his Music & Memory program is simple and elegant. Residents are given iPods filled with their own musical favorites—a soundtrack of their lives. Musical favorites tap deep memories not lost to dementia and can bring clients back to life, enabling them to feel like themselves again, to converse, socialize, and stay present. By talking with the resident and their friends and relatives, a personal playlist can be developed. When it isn't possible to get this information from a client or family member, the year a person was born can provide valuable clues.

Research has shown we remain emotionally attached to music that was popular during our adolescent and young adult years. The clinical reasons this music has therapeutic value relates to the areas of the brain involved in emotion, association, and long-term memory. These areas include the limbic system (the amygdala and hypothalamus) and the medial prefrontal cortex. These areas and the neural networks that link them can still be stimulated through the auditory pathways in people with Alzheimer's and dementia.

I contacted Dan Cohen to learn more about the program. He shared some talking points that might help convince a wary administrator to sign on for staff training to implement the program. He provided data from a study that showed the use of iPods enabling some facilities to remove patients from anti-psychotic medications.

Nothing happens quickly but after three years I succeeded, in part by securing matching funds, to bring the program to the Elkins Rehabilitation & Care Center.

Although the human voice and our connections as we sing together seem to provide the most therapeutic value, the iPod can fill a hole left when residents are alone and isolated.

I introduced the Music & Memory program at ERCC with iPods programmed for three of the residents: Margaret, who loves big band music; Estelle, whose agitation I hoped would abate with gentle harp stylings; and old-time country music for Hazel, who was one of the most disturbed and isolated of the residents.

Margaret tapped her toes and sang along... for a while... but then pulled off the headphones. They were bothering her and messing up her hairdo.

Estelle visibly delighted in the harp music, and was still aware of what was going on around her. She would pull the headset aside if some disturbance seemed to be in the offing, especially during the time of day when she asserted her authority as owner of the building. In this role, it was important for her to be in charge.

One day she took off her headphones and showed them to Arthur. "What do you call this thing?" she asked a passing nurse. After learning the answer she turned back to the other gentleman. "An iPod? It's an iPod, Arthur. Do you like music?"

"I like Johnny Cash," he replied.

Estelle approached me to ask if I could fix Arthur up with an iPod. This was a great sign. The music was working for her and she wanted to share it with others.

"That's my mamma's music!" Hazel's hard edged, strongly accented Appalachian voice floated across the room.

Nearly blind and approaching 100 years of age, Hazel has her eyes closed, tears streaming down her cheeks. Toes tapping. I know from my conversations with Hazel that hers has been a hard life, filled with poverty, alcoholism, and violence. I've seen her put up her fists, ready to take on an imaginary foe when someone accidentally bumps her wheelchair. Now the music has brought her back, enveloped in a musical memory of her mother's love. The music we associate with early childhood memories as well as the music of adolescence remain with us throughout our lives.

Whenever I see Mr. Shannon—Sonny—we have a Willy Nelson moment, invariably ending with a duet of "You Were Always on My Mind." His iPod is easy to program. I can also connect two iPods together so that Sonny and his wife, Esther, can listen together.

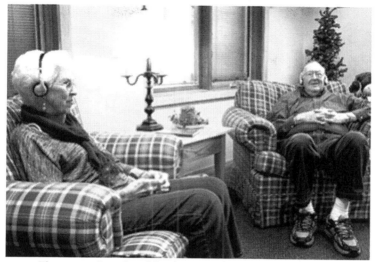

Gladys, another resident, walks into the room clutching her baby doll. She often believes that she is waiting for her husband to get home from the night shift, so she can go to her day job and he can take over child care. She is highly agitated this afternoon, her soft sobs becoming a keening, plaintive howl. I know I won't be able to put earphones on her, so I try to comfort her with synchronized singing, calibrating my voice with hers. When we're making music together our eyes lock. We are together in this drama. I switch our tune to "Amazing Grace," which she loves, and it eventually calms her restlessness. Maybe the next time she'll listen to it on an iPod.

Estelle has confided in me, "I miss Eddie terribly," she says, "but I'm still here and healthy. Oh, I know I'm forgetful, but I believe it would be satisfying to make something of the time I have left... to do something."

And thus, the ERCC Glee Club was formed.

All God's Critters got a place in the choir
Some sing low and some sing higher
Some sing aloud on the telephone wire
Some just clap their hands, or paws or
Anything they got now

This song by Bill Staines is a favorite with my group and another wonderful reminder that new tunes and melodies can be learned. Learned and *retained,* even with the limitations imposed by Alzheimer's disease.

This is what our daily music session looks like: I walk into the common room and begin the first song from "Singing in the Rain":

Good morning, good morning.
Did you dance the whole night through?
Good morning, good morning to you.

The residents jump into the song as though it's the last life-boat leaving the Titanic. Safe, secure, huddling together in this song, in this moment, they achieve calm and equality. They seem to be living inside the music.

I bring the group into a circle. Many people are in wheelchairs. One lucky resident will be awarded the honor of sitting with Toby.

We might start the session with "He's Got the Whole World in his Hands," or "The Hokey Pokey." These provide both vocal and physical warm-ups. We always joke at the end that it isn't even ten o'clock in the morning and we already know what it's all about. It's about "The Hokey Pokey."

On to "Oh What A Beautiful Morning" and another favorite from *Oklahoma*, "The Surry with the Fringe on Top."

Then it might be "My Favorite Things" or a seasonal song like "April Showers," "Over the River and Through the Woods," "Autumn Leaves" or "Easter Parade," "Sunny Side of the Street," "Blue Skies," or "Pennies from Heaven," or "Mockingbird Hill" and "She'll be Coming 'Round the Mountain."

Next our West Virginia songs: "West Virginia Hills," "West Virginia My Home," "Green Rolling Hills of West Virginia," and their favorite (not mine) "Country Roads," the Toby songs, lullabies, cowboy songs, patriotic numbers, favorite gospel numbers and hymns, then becoming traveling music for those who need to go to the bathroom or are being transported to physical therapy.

Hank Williams is a solid winner, because his songs reach across the generations. It's always great when nurses and nursing assistants can add their voices to the mix. We may not have a million tunes under our belt, but we have a reliable fifty in our repertoire. When not making our own music, I slip a CD in the player, trying to accommodate varied musical tastes.

Sometimes the results are surprising. While listening to "Don't Sit Under the Apple Tree with Anyone Else But Me," from a collection of WWII songs, the lyric "*till I come marching home*" prompts Ethel to start talking about her brothers and future husband returning from the war. This ignited memories in other listeners, and led to a lively discussion.

I often invite guest musicians to play for the residents. My husband Don's music is greatly enjoyed. We also have a flute player, Linda Wolfersheim, who joins us regularly, and once we even had a visit from a world class concert pianist, artist-in-residence at the local college. Jack Gibbons, whose performance venues include Carnegie Hall, was greatly amused and delighted when a resident informed him, "You have the *piano* in 'pianoforte' down pat, but perhaps your *forte* is too forte."

Inspired by his performance, I dressed Toby In *white tie and tail* and played a CD of George Gershwin's music followed by a screening of *Swing Time* with Fred Astaire and Ginger Rogers.

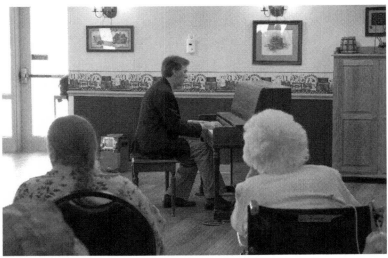

Figure 16: Jack Gibbons at the Elkins Rehabilitation & Care Center, 2011, with Ellen on the right in the front row. Photo by Grace Roy.

The residents feel acknowledged and appreciated when offered a private performance. Their graciousness reflects the good manners of an earlier era. Again, they are *my* teachers.

Two elderly visitors to the facility stirred my own musical memories and made me ponder what I would add to my personalized playlist.

I use Toby's office with the shiny new cabinet to store and program iPods for the Music & Memory program. Prime real estate though it is, it's still an airless, windowless room, and if you eat so much as a stale package of those orange-colored, faux cheese crackers, the smell lingers in the air for the next twenty-four hours.

While I work on playlists, Toby naps in his Amelia Earhart suitcase bed, dreaming perhaps of deer jerky. The sound of an accordion drifts across the hall from the large activity room. It sounds like the real deal—not a rerun of Lawrence Welk—so I've got to check it out. I scoop up Toby, cross the hall, and open the door to the activity room. I'm astounded to see two men, perhaps in their eighties, looking and sounding like they stepped out of a 1940's dance band and speaking like they hail from southwestern Pennsylvania. Polka music.

Mom will love this, I thought. I approached Trisha, the activity aid, who was hunkered over her chair, presenting plumber's butt and pulling on her split ends. She had never shown any interest in the musical groups visiting the facility whether jazz, flute ensembles, gospel singers, not even country. "How long will they be here?" I whisper.

"I dunno." she responds, looking up from the newspaper insert offering super deals on supersized subs.

"When did they start?"

"I dunno."

She's supposed to oversee this activity yet has only brought in a handful of residents. Reading my expression, I can tell she has some concern that I might *get her in trouble*. It is not a pleasant job for her. She

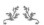

also doubles as a CNA—certified nursing assistant—a position requiring fewer course hours than it takes to become certified as a hairdresser in this state.

I tell her I want to know how long they'll be playing so I can decide if there's time to bring my mother over from the dementia unit.

"I dunno," she says again.

It's worth a try. I race down the hallway, Toby at my heels, through the double locked doors of the dementia unit, where I find Mom, sitting in her wheelchair with the sad old stuffed kitty on her lap, wearing one of the colorful pull-on skirts I've made for her. This is the one covered with tea cups.

I put Toby on her lap and begin steering the wheelchair toward the activity room.

"She loves polka music, she loves polka music, *sheee* loves polka music." I make up a sort of polka mantra as we careen down the hall. Dancing tea cups, dancing Pennsylvania tea cups, I sing to a polka beat.

"Where are you taking me?" she asks, with some measure of alarm.

"We're going to listen to polka music. You'll like it. It's *like FUN*," I say lamely, speaking louder now as we near the activity room.

I can hear the accordions. I wheel Mom close to the performers, but she's closed in on herself. She smiles wanly at kitty, then doubles over holding her near. Toby adjusts and finds his own space beside kitty.

I keep trying, shouting out things like, "MORE Polkas, WE HAVE A PENNSYLVANIA GIRL HERE!" Or did I say "Gal"? What's the matter with me? I don't talk like this.

I personally do not care for polka music, but these guys are good, really good. It's sweet, too, the way they

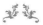

tell jokes between numbers, speaking in the vernacular of the era, dated, but sweet.

It's like a window back in time, a window back to my time, my early time. I've pretty much forgotten about Mom. I touch her back. She's safe. I'll return her to the dementia unit soon. I close my eyes as they fill with tears. I rarely cry anymore, but it would feel good to cry right now. It's not the right time, not appropriate so I stifle the flow keeping my eyes closed.

What's that they're playing? It's familiar, from someplace long ago and far away. I keep my eyes closed, forgetting my mother so close, but lost to me.

Another *mother* materializes, playing the upright piano in my grandparents' living room. I'm four-year-old Linda Jo, lying on the floor on the rug in the Old Stone house. My eyes are closed but with my mind's eye other senses amplify. I can smell the mixture of dust and mothballs as I feel the beat of the music pulsating through the floor boards.

"The last song you played," I shout over the drum machine. "What was it?"

I must repeat my question several times. They're pretty hard of hearing, but they're wonderful and they are *playing real good for free*. I love it! I love them! I love polka music! Maybe they'd come to the farm and play for my birthday. Finally, they hear me.

"The Blue Skirt Waltz," they say in unison. I notice how alike they are. They must be brothers, maybe twins.

Leaping to my feet, I break into what I think may be a polka. It feels right.

Mom holds up kitty, grins, nods her head in a knowing way and says, "Good!"

And it is.

At the end of the day, I go to Mom's room and sit by her bed. Nora is resting peacefully in the adjoining bed. Here Ellen is surrounded by a few well-loved stuffed cats. Her bed is covered with a feline themed comforter, a gift from a staff member. Her head is resting on a thrift store pillow, embellished with pansies and the word "Love." With excellent eyesight, reading being an overlearned behavior, she still likes to read words, and is in fact, fascinated by them. I've been leaving short messages on a whiteboard for years now. The message board allows her to hold onto the words. Exchanging short funny word messages and drawings is both entertaining and comforting.

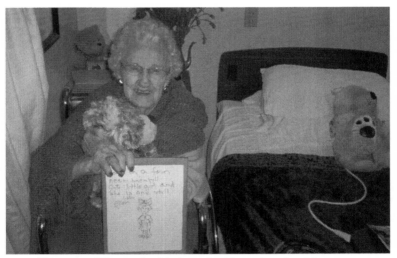

Figure 17: Ellen and whiteboard with my handwriting, 2012

She is less able to comprehend their meanings than she was a few months ago, though the fascination is still there. At the dentist's office last week, she read aloud: *"Payment must be rendered at the time of service unless prior arrangements have been made,"* repeatedly.

Sometimes her use of words and metaphor are poetic, like, "I love who you are. May I have the words?" she responds during a poetry session.

I don't know if she understands the meaning of these words. Yet of course she does, even if she doesn't *appear* to know that she is Ellen or Mrs. Zimmer, or even what a mother or daughter is. She doesn't have names for her stuffed cats, not that she can verbalize, though she is obviously attached to them. I try to keep items in her room simple, stimulating, but not cluttered. When she loses interest in a stuffed animal, it goes to the farm where it is adopted by the gentle poodle giant, J. Jasper Jones.

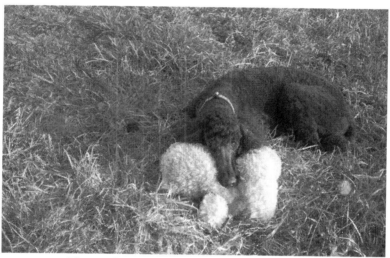

Figure 18: Jasper and adopted pink bear, 2014

Mom invariably comments on my clothing. "I like your shoes," she says, or, "That skirt looks really good on you. I like its blues."

She's resting now, with Toby, a fuzzy apricot ball at her feet. She opens her eyes as I softly play "John of

Dreams" on the dulcimer. I smile at her and whisper, "I love you." She nods and closes her eyes again.

I put down the dulcimer and begin writing in my notebook. I know the calm of this moment can be shattered at any time by a scream, an alarm, or a wandering resident entering the wrong room—this one.

I want to finish my notes, so I can scoop up Toby, do some late afternoon shopping and return to the farm.

Mom's awake again. She's trying to focus on the makeshift nametag I attached to my sweater when I left the official badge in the car.

"Linda?" she asks, holding her head to one side.

She's confused. I don't usually try to straighten out facts for her, but I'm so happy to hear her say my name that I respond with animation, "Yes, I'm Linda. I'm your daughter, you're my mom."

Still confused, she looks at me intently and says, "You have Linda?"

What does she mean? I understand that people with Alzheimer's often use the wrong verb tense.

"Yes, I have Linda," I respond, "and we will all take care of each other."

From the next bed I hear Nora's small voice ask, "And me too?"

"Yes, you too," I say.

"I'm glad to know that," Mom intones in a relaxed confident manner. "I didn't know that." Then she adds, "I like your dress!"

I recently watched the film, *Avatar*. When the characters say, "I see you," they are really saying, "I love you." I remember Fred Rogers and the song "There are Many Ways to Say I Love You." Really seeing

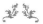

another person and allowing them to see you is the greatest gift you can give another person.

Music remains a life line for my mother. Unable to communicate with words, we hold hands and share a dance to a recording of "Old Flames Can't Hold a Candle to You."

"No one lights up my life like you do."

I lock eyes with her and mirror her movements. Her timing is as perfect as ever. Her light has shown in this world for 98 years, often illuminating my own path, yet I know it is fading now. Her joys: a satisfying meal involving ice cream, a pain free cozy nap with a well-loved stuffed cat. An appreciation of nature in a single fresh flower brought to her bedside or sitting in the sun in Toby's garden.

The days dwindle down to a precious few in September, *"...and these few precious days I'll spend with you..."*

Sometimes it seems like all life's big moments have a soundtrack or recurring theme. Leaving the nursing home after my mother Ellen McCay dies, the car radio is playing Nellie McCay singing "Every Time We Say Goodbye." Its haunting lyrics and chord change: *"How strange the change from major to minor every time we say goodbye,"* reminds me there have been many goodbyes before this final one, many shifts of mood and tempo in this journey. I'm filled with gratitude for them all.

The End

Epilogue

I developed the Playful Protocol to help my mother cope with the challenges of living with Alzheimer's disease. We found common ground in our mutual love of music, art and animals, while I discovered that human beings maintain their access to emotions and creativity for their entire lifespan.

Since the power of theatre saved me—a shy and awkward adolescent in a small town in West Virginia—the arts have continued to inspire, engage, and enrich my life. Through my attempt to help first my own mother and then others in a nursing home, I now understand I was also saving myself.

Oliver Sacks described being "musicked along" in a dramatic moment in his book, *A Leg to Stand On,* when he uses the power of music, singing and feeling the rhythm *of The Volga Boatman,* to push himself down a hill after sustaining injuries from being attacked by a bull. Perhaps this is too large a metaphor for my experience, but harnessing the power of music, art, drama and nature was key to my goal of maintaining active engagement for my clients and myself.

I played several roles on the nursing home stage:
- Arts therapist
- Ellen's daughter
- Toby, the therapy dog's mom

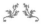

- Embedded investigative reporter and perhaps what I believed to be most important: advocate or *spy*.

Over the course of seven years, I morphed from the perky assurance of Nancy Drew to the mature sleuthing of Jessica Fletcher, to the invisibility and (hopefully) wisdom of an agilely aging Miss Marple.

Because the pat descriptions of individuals with Alzheimer's disease portraying them as victims and sufferers is so frequently employed, these people are often warehoused and forgotten while we have walks and fundraisers, waiting for the cure, hoping scientists find it before *we* develop the disease. This well-intentioned media hype confirms our worst fears and superstitions. People with Alzheimer's have disappeared along with their memories, we're told. "No use looking for them, better to stay away."

The Playful Protocol is not rocket science though it is grounded in scientific research. Many caregivers as well as arts therapists and healthcare professionals have long been aware anecdotally, of the positive impact that participation in the creative arts has on people's mood, cognitive vitality, and general sense of well-being.

Now because of technical advances giving scientists the ability to monitor brain activity in real time, we have the consilience of the creative arts and brain health.

It was once common belief that the human brain gradually lost neurons and became less able to function. We now know, given the right conditions, the adult human brain will continue to develop new brain cells, allowing even people with dementia, the possibility of creating new neural pathways, which can be facilitated through creativity and the arts. Participating in creative activities can challenge the older brain and induce the sprouting of new dendrites, thereby enhancing brain reserve. Brains of older adults tend to be more lateralized than younger brains, allowing more integration of left and right brain involvement. Lateralization of functioning changes with healthy aging, switching to bilateral patterns, bringing older adults processing resources to bear on a new task as a way of compensation. While nothing like a cure, the Playful Protocol can often bring people back, if only for a time.

When my mother died in 2015, I believed myself, despite mounting evidence to the contrary, to be working in a facility with a commitment to developing an enlightened memory care unit.

Instead it had become a locked unit for people with the most severe behavior problems.

As an arts therapist and advocate, I lobbied the administration to provide training from outside experts. They opted for online tutorials to educate staff in understanding the Alzheimer's disease process and provide tips on appropriate care. These courses could be completed by employees as they sat at a computer fielding cries for help and attention by the very residents they were being educated to care for.

I was heartsick. I had not succeeded in institutionalizing what I had seen with my own eyes, heard with my own ears, and touched with my heart and voice.

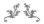

Then I remembered what Fred Rogers had said to children in times of trauma. "Look for the helpers." And there were many.

Some were the handful of dedicated nurses and nursing assistants who worked tirelessly for little monetary recompense or career status, to help meet the overwhelming physical and emotional needs of the residents. Family members who pitched in to help not only their own loved ones but other residents as well. Cleaning staff who went the extra mile to offer compassion along with fresh laundry. And the residents themselves as they looked after each other and strove to find simple gifts and honor the unique possibility of each new day.

As I spent time with the residents and my own mother, I was able to synchronize my clock with theirs—to live in the moment—their moment in time, playing with Toby, playing with words and music, Playing with Memory.

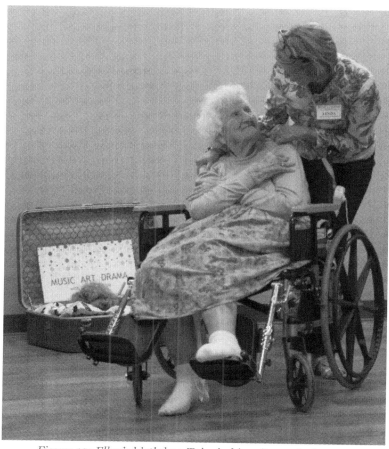

Figure 19: Ellen's birthday. Toby in his suitcase-bed, 2013.
Photo by Grace Roy.

Resources

Some of the resources that inspired me as I created The Playful Protocol:

Ackerman, Diane. *Deep Play.* Random House, 1999.

Halpern, Sue. *A Dog Walked into a Nursing Home.* Penguin Random House, 2013.

InDepthCrew. "Linda Zimmer - Marionette Puppetry and Expressive Arts Therapy," video: youtu.be/uMS3_T4pDzs

Marshall, Karrie. *Puppetry in Dementia Care: Connecting through Creativity and Joy.* Jessica Kingsley Publishers, 2013.

Music & Memory program. musicandmemory.org

New York Museum of Modern Art dementia program. moma.org

Oliver, James. *Contented Dementia.* Reprint edition. Vermillion, 2010.

Rise Up Singing, lyrics and guitar chords for over 1200 songs by Annie Patterson and Peter Blood. www.riseupandsing.org.

Rylant, Cynthia. *The Relatives Came.* Aladdin, 1993.

Sacks, Oliver. *Musicophilia: tales of music and the brain.* Alfred A. Knopf, 2007.

Therapy Dogs International. www.tdi-dog.org

Various poetry collections, art prints, and calendar art.

Song Resources

"All God's Critters Got a Place in the Choir" by Bill Staines, 1984.

"Hey, Good Lookin'. What Ya Got Cookin'?" Hank Williams, 1951.

"How Much is that Doggy in the Window?" lyrics by Bob Merrill, recorded by Patti Page, 1952.

"I'm Your Puppet" performed by Marvin Gaye and Tammi Terrell, 1966.

"In the Garden" by C. Austin Mills, 1913.

"Over the Rainbow" music by Harold Arlen and lyrics by Yip Harburg for *The Wizard of Oz*, performed by Judy Garland, 1939.

"Someone to Watch Over Me" music by George Gershwin and lyrics by Ira Gershwin for *Oh, Kay!*, recorded by Gertrude Lawrence, 1927.

"Stormy Weather" by Harold Arlen and Ted Koehler, performed by Ethel Waters, 1933.

Words and music to

Bloom and Sing

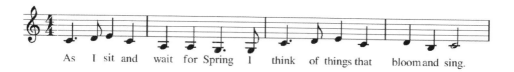

As I sit and wait for Spring I think of things that bloom and sing.

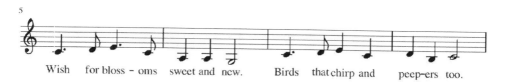

Wish for bloss - oms sweet and new. Birds that chirp and peep-ers too.

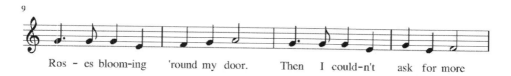

Ros - es bloom-ing 'round my door. Then I could-n't ask for more

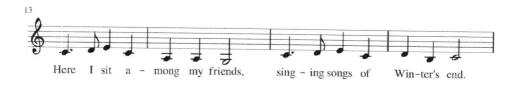

Here I sit a - mong my friends, sing - ing songs of Win-ter's end.

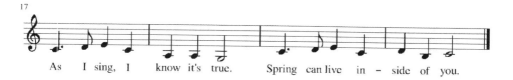

As I sing, I know it's true. Spring can live in - side of you.

Linda and Toby's

Blue Ribbon Maple Scones

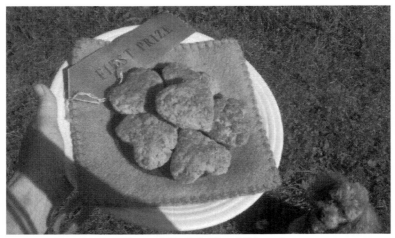

Figure 20: Toby and Linda's Blue Ribbon Scones, 2015

Great for people and dogs!
(Dogs will be happy with these a day or two after they're made, a little dry and crumbly.)

Preheat oven to 425 degrees.

Combine:
    1 cup whole wheat flour
    1 cup all-purpose flour
    1/3 cup brown sugar
    1 tablespoon baking powder
    1/2 teaspoon salt
    1/4 teaspoon cinnamon

Whisk 1 cup heavy cream with 1/4 cup maple syrup.

Stir dry and wet ingredients until just blended.

Knead against the side of the bowl several times and turn out onto a lightly floured surface. Divide dough in half and form two circles approximately 3/4" thick. Cut each circle into 8 wedges and place on ungreased baking sheet. Bake 12 to 15 minutes.

Make a glaze with confectioner's sugar and maple syrup to top scones.

Finger puppet template

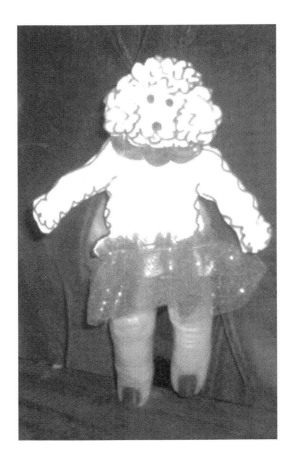

Create your own Toby finger puppet!

INSTRUCTIONS:

The design is printed at actual size. Permission granted to photocopy these pages for personal use.

Color with watercolors, crayons, acrylics, markers, etc., then attach fabric or ribbon or tulle (see example on page 23).

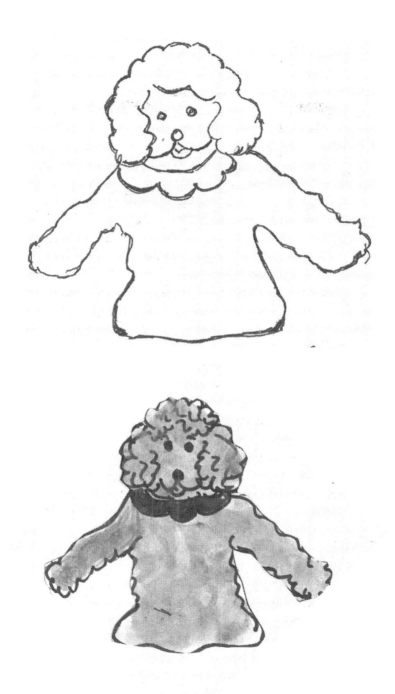

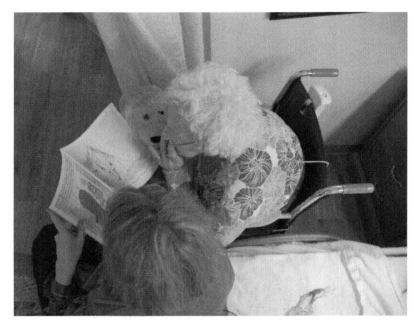

Figure 21: Linda and Ellen, 2010. Photo by Paul King.

About the Author

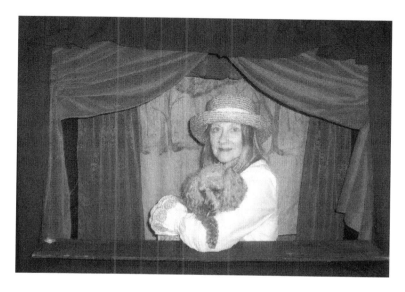

LINDA ZIMMER is a puppeteer, teaching artist, and expressive arts therapist.

After touring with The Lovelace Marionette Theater in Pittsburgh, she worked on *Mister Rogers' Neighborhood* where she created the puppets Betty Okanak Templeton, Turkey Express, and Old Goat.

She developed her own one-woman shows including *Lizzies Tune* about labor leader Mother Jones and *Eleanor's Garden* about Eleanor Roosevelt.

As Rita Saurus, a puppet character in the *Read America* program, she was interviewed on *Good Morning America* and appeared in public service announcements for the AARP.

The lovable and empathic dog puppet characters she created for children's hospitals helped kids share their feelings and cope with the trauma of hospitalization. Her work has been documented in national magazines.

Zimmer is co-author of the script for *Max and Nellies Journey with Grief,* a film funded by the Claude Worthington Benedum Foundation to help children cope with loss and grief.

She lives on an organic farm in the central mountains of West Virginia with her husband, Don Olson, at Blue Rock Farm where they produce maple syrup, rainbow trout, offer a U-pick blueberry patch, and maintain an heirloom apple orchard. She builds marionettes in her puppet studio while wrangling cats and poodles, and appears as Beatrix Potter in *Puppet Tales from Beatrix Potter.*

Playing with Memory was written while she and her therapy dog, Toby, made the daily thirty-mile trip on curving mountain roads to the town of Elkins, WV, to provide expressive arts and pet therapy to residents of a nursing home.

55845731R00071

Made in the USA
Middletown, DE
18 July 2019